Sisters on a Journey

Sisters
on a Journey

Portraits of American Midwives

Penfield Chester

Photography by Sarah Chester McKusick

Rutgers University Press
New Brunswick, New Jersey, and London

Library of Congress Cataloging-in-Publication Data

Chester, Penfield, 1955–
    Sisters on a journey : portraits of American midwives / Penfield
Chester ; photography by Sarah Chester McKusick.
        p.   cm.
    Includes bibliographical references and index.
    ISBN 0–8135–2407–5 (alk. paper). —ISBN 0–8135–2408–3 (pbk. : alk.
paper)
        1. Midwives—United States.   2. Midwifery—United States.
    3. Midwives—United States—Pictorial works.   4. Midwifery—United
    States—Pictorial works.   I. Title.
    RG950.C47   1997
    618.2'0233'0973—dc21   97-7711
                                                                                 CIP

British Cataloging-in-Publication information available

Text copyright © 1997 by Penfield Chester
Photographs copyright © 1997 by Sarah Chester McKusick; except photograph of
Sister Angela Murdaugh © 1997 by Jana Flores-Jon and photographs of Faith
Gibson, Toni House, and Candace Whitridge © 1997 by Penfield Chester.

All rights reserved

No part of this book may be reproduced or utilized in any form or by any means,
electronic or mechanical, or by any information storage and retrieval system, without
written permission from the publisher. Please contact Rutgers University Press,
Livingston Campus, Bldg. 4161, P.O. Box 5062, New Brunswick, New Jersey
08903. The only exception to this prohibition is "fair use" as defined by U.S.
copyright law.

Manufactured in the United States of America

618.2
C525

To all of my sisters in MANA, who strive to keep the essence of midwifery alive today, and to Ginny Miller and Liza Ramlow, two midwives in my community who have reached across the gap that threatens to separate the branches of midwifery. Even though as nurse-midwives their educational path and place of practice are very different from those of the midwives in my homebirth community, they have offered support and friendship as we strive to be united in our service to birthing women.

Contents

Acknowledgments

I want first to thank all the midwives interviewed here, both for sharing their time with me and for allowing me to share their stories with others. My desire is to have their voices heard outside the arena of midwifery as well as for midwives to hear each others' voices and opinions.

For leading me into midwifery in the first place, I thank Suzanne Arms. Her critique of the medical approach to birth and the powerful vision of a better way she articulated in her 1975 book *Immaculate Deception* were a tremendous influence. A number of other writers have helped me to clarify issues surrounding midwifery: Elizabeth Davis, Robbie Davis-Floyd, Raymond DeVries, Ina May Gaskin, Barbara Katz Rothman, Brigitte Jordan, and Judy Luce, to name a few. For solutions, I acknowledge the inspiration given to me by Eugene DeClercq, the Interorganizational Work Group's Vision Statement, the Women's Institute for Childbearing Policy paper, the midwives of Ontario and New Zealand, and finally the Midwives' Alliance of North America (MANA), whose inclusive quality is its strongest appeal and greatest challenge.

A number of women helped me transcribe, edit, and proofread the manuscript: Cynthia Battle, Eunice Bravmann, Karen Feiden, Jackie Meadows, Terri Nash, Lucinda Proctor, Suzi Voutselas, and Gene Zeiger. And I'd like to thank all those who nudged me, egged me on, propped me up in the long lesson of "how to finish" . . . particularly Margaret Blanchard, Deb Martin, Jackie Meadows, and my Canadian cousins. It was a group effort

that brought this book to light. Special thanks to Elizabeth Withnall for acting as interpreter during my interview with Jesusita Aragon.

I especially want to thank Robbie Davis-Floyd for her inspiring vision
and for her constant encouragement and patience.

In the personal realm, I want to thank my sister Sarah, who kept encouraging me as I slowly but doggedly finished the project (I would get a
prize for endurance rather than speed). I also want to thank my husband and
son, who had to endure my preoccupied state of mind for many weeks during
the writing. Sally Boutiette, with her skill in acupressure, her wonderful ability to listen, and her gentle, humorous presence, helped so much during the
last long haul. And finally, thanks to Marilyn Middleton, who helped me to
balance the amount of time spent in my frontal lobe with getting me back
down into my body with African dance.

Sisters on a Journey

Introduction

Midwifery is one of the world's oldest professions. Women have always attended other women in childbirth; even today the majority of babies come into the world through the hands of a midwife. Yet in the United States and Canada, midwifery was almost eradicated. The survival and current revival of American midwifery has been a direct result of midwives' connection to and identification with the women they serve. This bond has always been key to the practice of midwifery and spurred one of the first recorded acts of civil disobedience. As told in the Bible, Hebrew midwives resisted a royal order to kill firstborn sons; they refused and "saved the children alive."

When asked who I am or what I do, today I choose to answer that I am a midwife. My chosen profession is more than a job—it is an attitude, a philosophy, a heritage that sometimes fills me with a sense of honor and at other times feels like a burden. The very word *midwife*—"with woman"—evokes a sense of relationship, a definition of self in relation to another. I was drawn to midwifery because I wanted to be with women during the incredible process of pregnancy and birth. Later I found myself also drawn to midwives. I met midwives whose educational and cultural backgrounds were very different from my own and became curious about their stories and experiences. I wanted to know why they had taken up this calling, one that requires them to set their lives aside for a baby's unpredictable arrival. I wanted to know what gives them the courage and conviction to face life and death as each birth unfolds. I wanted to learn why they choose to attend births in the

1

face of physicians' hostility and, in many states, prosecution. I wanted to understand how they can practice in so many different ways, yet all claim with equal right the name of *midwife*.

The inspiration for this collection of portraits came from the close connection that my sister Sarah and I developed as a result of birth. I had attended her three births as her midwife, and she had come to some births with me as a photographer. Being with Sarah as she birthed her three daughters illuminated for me the sisterly essence of midwifery. It was Sarah who suggested that we embark on a joint creative journey to document the lives of midwives, one that would combine her interest in portraiture with my work in midwifery.

As I interviewed the women whose stories appear in this book, my own role as a midwife was ever present, not only because I share the same occupation as those I interviewed, but also because I was able to use skills developed through midwifery practice to build mutual trust, allowing for intimacy and for full, free expression to emerge in their stories. And as a midwife and an interviewer, I have had to ask myself again and again: Why have I undertaken this project? Who are these other women who have chosen—or been chosen—for this work, and how do their paths and choices differ from mine? As I look into the eyes and hearts of these women and listen to their voices, I strain to hear what is theirs and what is my own. Entering their lives, I receive a sense of their individuality and how it mixes into the pool of ancient wisdom of women serving women in childbirth. The threads of their stories link them to generations of past and future midwives. The questions I have asked other midwives I now ask myself.

I will share some of my history so that the nature of the lens through which the other midwives' stories are told will be clearer. My portraits of midwives are subjective, and I wish them to be so. They represent a give-and-take between the woman who created the portrait and the woman portrayed—an interplay as active as what I experience in the practice of midwifery.

Midwife as Self:
The Sisterly Art of Being with Woman

Emerging from a family of four sisters and an extended family of strong women, I came to midwifery with a feminist, woman-centered perspective. My energy in midwifing is a sisterly energy—the quality of being there, with

the loving teasing of sisters, the playfulness, the intimacy of knowing each other's secrets. From this background comes the ability to nurture and support each other when dealing with physical and emotional pain. Along with all the family quirks and squabbles and underlying tensions present as I grew up, there has always been support and unwavering love, which has fostered fierce independence and creativity in my own life. From my extended family in Canada, I learned the importance of connection, and I can see how our love and respect for the wild influences my beliefs about birth.

I was first attracted to birth when after college I worked on a farm and watched animals give birth. I saw that birth works well as a natural process and that animals only occasionally need assistance from attendants and rarely require further medical help from veterinarians. I studied movement therapy in college, developing a particular interest in the mind–body connection and its relationship to a woman's personal identity and empowerment—issues that became the backdrop for my interest in birth. I participated in what were then called "consciousness-raising groups" organized by the Boston Women's Health Book Collective and in women's self-help health groups, learning to do speculum exams and self breast exams. While I was pursuing this interest in women's health and working in a family-planning clinic, a friend invited me to her homebirth class. She graduated from the class—and I still haven't! Within a year, I went straight from childbirth education training to studying midwifery in a Boston program organized by two lay midwives, and followed that with an informal apprenticeship.

Although I had never conceived of working in what our culture defines as a medical field, I found myself drawn to help women reclaim birth as a bodily and social process in which women were respected, even honored. My desire was not to save or protect babies as much as to be *with women*, and by being with them to help them be healthy, happy mothers who would in turn support healthy babies. Doing so in this culture and time has required and given me the privilege of learning many technical, quasi-medical skills, but these skills are not my focus. My strength lies in the relationship I have with women, which I see as a sisterly connection. Attending my own sisters' births has shown me that my way of being with laboring women is similar to the way I am with my family. I use humor, story-telling, and comforting touch with women in labor. I try to adapt to their rhythms and blend with their energy. I draw on a calming voice and presence in myself to ease their fear. I can, however, become abrupt and even bossy when a problem calls for immediate action.

When I started my midwifery training in 1980, I could see a need for trained midwives to attend the women and families who were choosing homebirths. One route was to become a nurse and then a certified nurse-midwife (CNM). But I did not want to become a nurse—I felt nursing would deny me the background needed to help in a normal, healthy process. Moreover, in my state at that time, certified nurse-midwives were prohibited by law from attending homebirths. This left only lay midwives to serve families who wanted homebirths. The legal standing of our practice was ambiguous until 1985, when a federal court judge ruled that lay midwifery is legal in Massachusetts. Ironically, the judge ruled at the same time that the state nursing board could forbid nurses from attending homebirths. The result was that, in Massachusetts, anyone except a nurse could attend a homebirth. In the face of this absurdity, I was glad I had chosen to become a lay midwife.

Midwifery has a long tradition of training through apprenticeship. Although American society today primarily respects and relies on institutionally based education, apprenticeship has great value as a tool for passing on the intricate knowledge and art of midwifery. Midwifery demands creative thinking when decisions need to be made and the confidence to be there "with women" during prenatal care and labor. But the near disappearance of American midwifery in previous decades broke the tradition of apprenticeship: there was no longer a clear-cut model of what apprenticeship should or could be. So, following my year of formal study, I had to invent an apprenticeship for myself. I found I was well served by the independent work and creative thinking emphasized throughout my undergraduate years at Hampshire College. Over the next five years, I attended births with a number of different midwives, learning from the differences in their style and primarily from the experience of birth itself. Eventually I had my own homebirth practice. Nevertheless, I always attended births with other midwives, working side-by-side. Over time, we developed a group practice.

When I gave birth to my son, I experienced the tension of wanting to create a positive birth experience yet having to be open to and learn from whatever happens. I had often amused myself (and kept myself awake on long rides home from births in the middle of the night) with fantasies of whom I'd want to have with my husband and me during our birth. But when I went into labor almost eight weeks before our son was due, his prematurity meant going far away to a hospital that had an intensive-care unit for babies. I had to let go of all my previous ideas about my birth and pay attention to the immediate lessons. I discovered how important it is for the family to be considered

and worked with as an integral unit after a birth. I longed to perch like a nesting hen on my son's incubator and keep him close to my body and breath. What I instinctively felt then has since been recognized as valuable: "kangaroo care" is a philosophy of keeping premature babies skin-to-skin with their mothers, who are far better than machines at providing warmth, comfort, stimulation, and care.

I also came to appreciate the importance of humor in labor—I'll never forget the slow March fly buzzing through the delivery room, hovering over my body as the resident and nurse looked on, distraught with keeping their gloves and the "sterile field" uncontaminated. The rebellious fly gave me just the right belly laugh to let go and push my little one out.

I experienced the vulnerability of a new parent, the fear of being in an institution whose values and ways of looking at things are different from my own. I learned how different hospital birth is from being at home. My experience up until then was primarily homebirth, so I felt—even in the middle of it all—that this experience was going to help me be a better midwife. Afterward, I ruefully remembered saying during my pregnancy that I should visit an NICU (neonatal intensive-care unit) to round out my midwifery training, not thinking it would be with my own baby. And I learned how, when a planned homebirth abruptly ends up transferred to a hospital, a midwife (in this case my own midwifery partner) can help restore the sense of connection during the postpartum period.

Natural birth does not necessarily mean a happy birth, for nature is not always kind. There came a time, after attending some difficult births, when I questioned whether I could continue to face the stress and possible heartbreak of attending births. Initially I had been drawn to this work by the power of women in their glory of giving birth to precious newborns, not out of a sense of responsibility to protect birth from death. I had to face the shadow side of midwifery, of death being the soul sister to birth. I could feel the power of fear as it threatened to choke the power of love. The fear of blame, of not knowing enough, of not making the right decision at the right time—ultimately the fear of death—closed in on me. I decided to make death a friend, or at least an ally. I undertook volunteer hospice training so I could spend more time reflecting on death. Rather than ignore or run from it, I learned to acknowledge its presence and to listen to my feelings of love rather than fear. I am always shaken by the experience of having to resuscitate a baby or of stopping the life-threatening loss of blood during a bad hemorrhage. These are the times we can see how closely the lines of birth and death

are intertwined, and I look inward and outward for the energy of love and the strength of faith that it takes to keep doing this soul-wrenching work. My desire to interview other midwives was, in part, a personal need to hear how others cope with the emotional demands and fears that birth can bring up. Hearing other midwives' stories is a source of renewal, a way of nurturing the spiritual faith that many midwives consider crucial to this work.

The Midwifery Model Contrasted with the Medical Model of Childbirth

I am an avid reader: my initial interest in midwifery came in part from reading *Immaculate Deception,* in which Suzanne Arms so graphically portrayed the plight of American women in childbirth. I supplemented my experiential education of attending births by reading anything on midwifery and birth I could get my hands on. I read *Williams Obstetrics,* the bible of obstetrical texts, as well as Ina May Gaskin's alternative classic *Spiritual Midwifery,* and all the birth and midwifery journals I could find. Twelve years later, at Vermont College I continued my education with a master's program in women's studies with a focus in midwifery, in which I studied the history of midwifery, midwifery educational theory and practice, and the anthropology of birth.

As I sought to understand the forces affecting midwifery as it tries to survive in this country and to explain the appeal that attending homebirths has for me as a midwife, I turned to the work of many social scientists and birth activists (for example, Arms 1975, 1995; Arney 1982; Rothman 1982, 1989; Davis-Floyd 1992, 1994; Martin 1987; Sullivan and Weitz 1988). Barbara Katz Rothman and Robbie Davis-Floyd, in particular, illuminated for me the key differences between the ways obstetricians and midwives look at childbirth. Drawing from sociology, anthropology, the history of medicine, and women's studies, Rothman and Davis-Floyd articulated what we homebirth midwives know to be true in our hearts and from our experiences.

Rothman first described the medical and midwifery models of birth in 1982; a decade later, Davis-Floyd (1992) developed the idea further, using the terms *technocratic* and *holistic* to differentiate the two models, and defining *technocracy* as a society organized around an ideology of technological progress. In the technocratic model of birth, the body is seen as a machine defined by its separate pieces rather than as an integrated whole. In this view, pregnancy and birth are mechanical processes that are all too apt to break

down. The obstetrician in the hospital has the authority, the special tools, and the superior know-how to diagnose and fix the problems even before they happen, which is done by treating each stage of labor, as well as each body part, as separate and discrete. Even the language of medicine objectifies the woman and separates her into parts and from her baby. She does not give birth, but is "delivered" by the obstetrician; in one out of every five births in American hospitals, she will be "sectioned." Doctors are the supreme technicians who direct, manage, and control labor, and who maintain responsibility for the outcome. Their actions are driven by a belief in the supremacy of technology over nature and the truth of biomedical science. They base their actions on objective, measurable "facts" and view the process of labor as a means of bringing out a product—a healthy baby—separate from the integrated needs of mother and child. Indeed, separation is the basic principle underlying the technocratic model of birth (Davis-Floyd 1992).

When a woman gives birth within the medical model, she needs to fit into the institution's routine, and her labor has to fit into the parameters of what is considered normal. Her birth is "managed," or directed, rather than allowed to unfold in its own unique way. The unequal power relationship between patient and doctor means that the woman often must passively accept the physician's management of her labor and birth. In turn, physicians will maintain separation from patients: their touch will be impersonal, as in the routine cervical exams they will perform, often without asking the woman's permission. Having to use intrusive, sometimes hurtful touch in medical interventions (for example, in starting IVs, catheterizing, or giving injections) heightens a physician's impulse, ingrained throughout medical training, to separate or distance doctor from patient. Lacking any sort of trust in the normalcy of birth, most physicians believe that they must perform such interventions in almost every labor.

In contrast, the holistic model holds that birth is a normal, woman-centered process in which mind and body are one and that, in the vast majority of cases, nature is sufficient to create healthy pregnancy and birth. The midwife is seen as a nurturer. Her experiential and emotional knowledge is gained from an intimate relationship developed by providing ongoing care to a woman throughout her pregnancy and birth and after the baby is born. This connection is considered to be of more value than technical knowledge; indeed, connection is the basic principle underlying the holistic midwifery model. A midwife knows that a woman's uterus is not separate from the rest of her being; that emotional issues, stress, and fear can affect the process of

labor; and that attention to such issues will often do more to ensure a healthy labor than any machine. Because the midwife sees birth as an activity that women do to bring forth new life, during which authority and responsibility remain intrinsic to the woman, the midwife does not take over and "manage" the birth but rather serves as facilitator, guardian, and guide (Davis-Floyd 1992).

Of course, these models do not specifically describe the beliefs or actions of any particular individual, either doctor or midwife. A doctor can practice the art of midwifery, just as a midwife can attend birth in a medical manner. Nonetheless, the models do succeed in highlighting the profound differences between obstetrician-managed birth and midwife-attended birth. As the portraits of individual midwives show, the practices and beliefs of individual midwives stretch across the whole tension-filled spectrum that ranges between these two models of birth.

From intimate experience, both as a mother and a midwife, I know the difference between homebirth and institutionally based medical birth. As midwives, we view ourselves as guests in a woman's home, trying to fit in without disturbing the atmosphere she has created, to blend with the family. We are conscious about bringing the tools of the trade into a situation without bringing attention to them—unwrapping the noisy paper around instruments when the woman has gone to take a walk or a bath, trying to make changes in the environment in ways so as not to disturb her work. We slide the portable oxygen tank behind a door to be prepared and yet to avoid drawing the family's attention to it. We try to keep the woman as the focus, the central actor, and not get carried away with the business of our role as caregiver, or making her self-conscious by busily taking notes. Primarily we need to *be there*, observing, supporting, taking the lead when change is needed; being firm, clear, encouraging, patient, and kind; and giving her the connection of loving touch.

Eyes connecting, hearts connecting, we assure the woman that we are here, that her work in labor is powerful and good and will bring her baby. Our soothing words and gentle touch serve her as cues for relaxation. Occasionally we find that a stern, clarifying voice is best for giving the woman the reassurance and encouragement she needs when she reaches what she feels are her limits. And we use touch for comfort and guidance, not only to probe for information—applying counterpressure on her back; pressing on her vaginal muscles to give her a kinesthetic map of where to relax and to show her viscerally the place to push through, down into and through the birth canal;

and supporting her perineum as the vulva swells and opens to release the baby. Our touch ranges from the gentle stroking of her forehead to deep massage on her trembling thighs, which quake with the power of birth. Touching the woman in those ways, we as midwives are touched as well. When our hearts are opened in the intimate relationship of birth, we receive this opening as a gift from the mother who labors to bring forth into this world the continuation of our species.

The connection we have with women and the birth process (which would not be available if we maintained an uninvolved professional distance) can affect us personally on a soul level. I am rewarded for whatever I give by seeing the growth and change in women and families, by witnessing the miracle of a newborn baby, and by learning to incorporate some of those ways of being into my own life.

Three Strands of Midwifery

My bond with the individual women I serve as a midwife makes me fervently determined to help midwifery survive, so that women can give birth in honor and with respect. Midwifery in North America was almost lost, in part because midwives did not organize quickly enough to build community and communication either among themselves or with the women who want midwives to be with them at birth. The threats to midwifery have come from two directions: the first being the opposition of the medical establishment and its allies, and the second being conflicts among ourselves about what we are, how we learn, and how we practice.

Midwives today span the spectrum of practice in a way that is unique among callings—it is hard to think of another profession or group that is so diverse. Even as we resist others' attempts to define and restrict us, we have to be wary of doing the same to ourselves. Sheila Kitzinger has pointed out the danger of adopting one stereotype over another:

> Midwives today are not quite sure who they are or what they want to be. And maternity care systems often seem even less certain about the role and function of midwives. . . . The contrast between the stereotypes of the romantic and super-professional images implies a dichotomy between caring on the one hand and expertise on the other, as if midwives can only be caring if they are purely intuitive and can only exercise the intellect when using expensive and complicated machines to intervene in a natural physiological process. This polarity is typical of much thinking in obstetrics, as if the caregiver must choose

between the old "bedside manner," with its connotations of the bearded nineteenth-century doctor watching over the patient dying of pneumonia, and in contrast, the surgeon-savior, intellectually vigorous, emotionally detached, powerful to control women's wayward bodies. . . . The polarization of images of the midwife is not just inaccurate. It is dangerously wrong. For the midwife cannot be skilled without being caring. She cannot be truly caring without being skilled. (Kitzinger 1988:8)

If we let our differences rather than our commonalities define us, it will be difficult to work together. In midwifery, we can look at all the subcategories—nurse-midwife, community midwife, traditional midwife, Christian midwife, lesbian midwife—and if our gaze lingers on the qualifier rather than *midwife,* we can be pulled apart. If we start with the awareness and recognition that each of us is a unique individual with a distinct history, however, then we can move into community. It is what we have in common that brings us close: the sharing of breath, the sharing of birth and death. When we can join hands in a circle with those who practice differently, who come from different cultures and believe in gods or religions different from our own, then we can go forward in this work together.

To understand how we got to this point and to understand the lives of the midwives portrayed in this book, it is important to look at the paths American midwifery has taken, from past to present.

Grand Midwives: The Unbroken Strand to the Past

Until the early decades of the twentieth century, midwives were the primary caregivers in the vast majority of American births. Colonial midwives like Martha Ballard cared for hundreds of women during their careers (Ulrich 1991). Immigrant midwives brought rich stores of knowledge and diverse birthing traditions with them to America. Pioneer women became midwives out of necessity, caring for women on the ever-expanding frontier. But by the 1930s, physicians had replaced midwives as primary caregivers for birthing women, the hospital had replaced the home, and many strands in the tapestry of American midwifery were broken.

But some were not. Today, the grand midwife represents the original and traditional American midwife. She has carried on the legacy of midwifery as it was handed down to her in the form of personal apprenticeship by her mother, aunt, grandmother, or other older, respected woman in her lineage.

She is the First Nations midwife chosen by her elders to serve the community, the African American midwife of the South who incorporated traditions of Africa into her practice of midwifery, and the *partera* of the Southwest, carrying on the ways and beliefs of the Hispanic communities she serves.

These traditional midwives, who learned their trade from individual women who went before them or sometimes simply by attending births, represent the end of an era. Unlike independent midwives and nurse-midwives, grand midwives practiced in accordance with the values and beliefs of their communities, without self-consciously comparing themselves with the dominant medical model of childbirth:

> Midwifery offers a unique look at women's culture outside the realm of men, one that evolved from and was framed by the needs of women. Midwifery is an institution that virtually precedes male culture, as opposed to reacting to it; so its history is a uniquely positive one. (Susie 1988:72)

Not surprisingly, grand midwives in the United States have felt the unrelenting hostility of the medical establishment even more than other midwives have. Much of their collective lineage of midwifery wisdom and lore was lost as restrictive legislation passed in state after state during the middle decades of this century barred them from practice and thus prevented them from sharing their heritage with younger apprentices (Campbell 1946; Buss 1980; Susie 1988; Logan 1989; Holmes 1990; Smith and Holmes 1996).

We are lucky that some traditional midwives have managed to preserve and publish their individual stories. One grand midwife from Alabama, Onnie Lee Logan, felt she was going to burst if her story were not told. Her overwhelming desire not to die without telling her story brought her together with an English professor who took down her autobiography (Logan 1989). Onnie Lee was given the Sage Femme Award by the Midwives' Alliance of North America (MANA) in 1989, and along with it, the opportunity to share her years of midwifery experience with other midwives before she died in 1995. The story of traditional Hispanic American midwife Jesusita Aragon has been captured, thanks to a minister, in the book *La Partera* (Buss 1980). Gladys Milton, a grand midwife in Florida, recounted her life in detail in *Why Not Me Lord?* (Bovard and Milton 1993). I had the privilege of interviewing both Jesusita Aragon and Gladys Milton for this book.

Some native American midwives have held on to and passed down their traditions. Others have sought additional knowledge, like Toni House, the

indigenous midwife I interviewed, who received instruction from her traditional elders and also trained in El Paso with independent midwives. She is an example of the blending of the traditional and the contemporary. This blend is also seen in Navajo grand midwife Faye Knoki, who was honored with MANA's Sage Femme Award in 1993 and is now handing down her traditional knowledge to her daughter Ursula. Ursula, as a nurse-midwife, can then merge current medical knowledge with traditional knowledge—a thoroughly postmodern phenomenon (Davis and Davis-Floyd 1996). When Faye was honored by MANA, Ursula spoke about her mother, describing how she learned from her the sacredness of birth, the connection of mother and child, and the special relationship between the midwife and the birthing woman.

The gradual elimination of grand midwives has been going on for years. The public health department of Florida, for example, saw these midwives only as a necessary evil. Once physicians could be enlisted to provide care to indigent communities, the grand midwives were considered a public menace (Susie 1988). In an advertising campaign during the 1930s and 1940s, the medical establishment strove to portray the grand midwife as "dirty," "ignorant," "a boozer," even "evil" (Susie 1988).

This picture of moral degradation was a far cry from the reputation grand midwives held in their own communities. There, the midwife's moral character went hand-in-hand with her work; it was one of her most important attributes and earned her the deepest respect. Midwives were sources of knowledge, not only about childbirth, but also about child rearing and general health. Regarded as social and spiritual counselors for the community, they were often given the highest places of honor within the church. These women attributed their gifts to God for calling them to their practice and guiding them to do the right thing (Susie 1988). Onnie Lee Logan tells a story of resuscitating a baby at one of the first births she attended, even though she had never been taught by the other midwife how to do it:

> You know why I did that? I asked God to he'p me to bring that baby
> to life if life was in it and He gave me the power to do it. I learned
> then who to depend on from that. That's what I did and that boy's
> married and got a house full of childrens. . . . No ma'am I hadn't been
> taught how to do that. I progressed that outa my mind. My own
> mind. There was a higher power and God gave me wisdom. Mother-
> wit, common sense. Wisdom came from on high. (Logan 1989:89)

But that combination of motherwit, faith, and skill could not prevail against red tape. In one of Debra Anne Susie's interviews with the grand midwives of Florida, a daughter describes how her mother, after attending the births of thousands of babies, was forcibly retired:

> You can't beat the system when you got the doctors out there saying do this, and then you got the nurse out there saying do this. No one is giving you feedback as to *why* it's happening, but you see it happening. It got to the place that Mother's ward was just catching dust, and I seen the time the calendar was just lined *up* with babies being born. . . . She just got to the place where she sat there and she looked at her equipment—no deliveries, no one coming. And she got, well, I would say, at first, she got a little angry about it. This type of thing, someone killing your career, is just like killing some member of the family that's real close. (Susie 1988:91)

The public health department also tried to make Gladys Milton retire, but she fared better: with the support of the Florida independent midwives and clients who were lawyers and knew how to fight the system, she won in court to preserve her practice (Bovard and Milton 1993).

These midwives were run out of practice on the belief that doctors have the knowledge and expertise to save women and babies from the hazards of childbirth in the midwives' hands. The midwife who grieved the demise of her practice claims in Susie's interview that she had very few stillbirths in her thirty years of service, and lost only one mother after the mother was in the hospital with a doctor attending to her (Susie 1988). The blame for infant mortality was unjustly put on these midwives—who had, considering the general health of the population and the limited resources (both physical and educational) available to them, very good outcomes.

Certainly, some of the lifesaving skills of surgery and the discovery of antibiotics to counter infection gave the medical profession new tools to deal with problems of childbirth. However, this technical and chemical prowess was brought to bear on all births rather than just the problem births and was intentionally used to negate the wisdom already existing within the heritage of midwifery. If physicians and public health departments had decided to work *with* the midwives, empowering them as front-line practitioners who could rely on physicians as a support system for women and babies with medical problems, a very different picture of health care would have emerged. So much money would have been saved, and the grand midwives, rather than

silently slipping away unacknowledged, would have proudly trained apprentices to blend their valuable midwifery knowledge with the newer medical insights and thus to carry on their accumulated expertise. Onnie Lee Logan observed that racism as illustrated by the disrespect shown to black families by the white medical profession precluded mutual understanding and cooperation between the two approaches to childbirth. The combined forces of racism and the need of the emerging medical profession to glorify itself as the cutting edge of modernity disallowed any such integration of thought. As a result, much of the grand midwife's expertise died with her.

Certified Nurse-Midwives

Nurse-midwives are unique in the field of midwifery in that they are trained in two professions: nursing and midwifery. The nurse-midwife is first trained in nursing and subsequently receives additional training as a midwife. "Nurse-midwifery is comprised of education in two disciplines that also incorporate components of a third discipline—medicine, specifically normal obstetrics, gynecology and neonatal medicine. . . . Nurse-midwifery is not totally nursing, not totally midwifery, and not medicine; it is a unique profession in its own right" (Varney 1987:4).

Historically, nurse-midwives entered midwifery through the public health model of nursing. They saw attendance at childbirth as part of bringing health care to the underserved populations of the rural and urban poor. One of the earliest nurse-midwives, Mary Breckinridge, created the Frontier Nursing Service by training midwives to attend births and give primary health care to families in Appalachia. She was educated in England and saw the usefulness of combining midwifery with public health nursing for families who had no other access to health care. The reduction in both infant and maternal mortality from this innovative service was remarkable (Breckinridge 1981).

In 1931 the Maternity Center in New York created the first formal educational program for nurse-midwives, the Lobenstine Midwifery School, which combined obstetrical nursing with education like that received by European midwives. Nurse-midwives were hired by public health departments in the South during the civil rights era and provided primary health care along with attending births. They also set up birth centers in the Southwest and in New York to help alleviate problems created by the lack of public health care available to the poor.

Certified nurse-midwives (CNMs) did not move into the arena of care-giving within private institutions until the early 1970s, when they began to attend the normal births of healthy, middle-class women. For the first time they became a threat to obstetricians, who had not minded the practice of nurse-midwifery as long as it remained part of the public health sector. Today, nurse-midwives work in all settings—hospitals, birth centers, and homes—and serve all types of populations. Approximately five thousand now practice in all states—more than 95 percent of them work in the hospital setting, giving care to normal and high-risk women; the rest work in free-standing birth centers or attend homebirths of low-risk women.

At first, the National Organization of Public Health Nurses established a section for nurse-midwives. Later nurse-midwives created their own organization, the American College of Nurse-Midwives (ACNM), which developed standards of education and practice, accreditation of educational programs, and a national certification exam (Varney 1987).

The relationship among nurse-midwifery, nursing, and the American College of Obstetricians and Gynecologists (ACOG) has often been rocky. This is not surprising, considering that a CNM's right to practice is tied into issues of power over collaborative or backup medical care and issues of competition and control. The agreement between the ACNM and ACOG establishes guidelines for nurse-midwifery practice with backup or consultation arrangements; it sets up a relationship by which nurse-midwives work in collaboration with obstetricians/gynecologists using mutually agreed-upon protocols (Varney 1987).

Nurse-midwives have argued that their combination of skills and collaboration with physicians makes their practices uniquely safe; and indeed the safety and satisfactoriness of the care that nurse-midwives provide has been extensively researched and documented (Goer 1995; Rooks 1997).

By defining themselves as unique, nurse-midwives worked to separate themselves from other midwives and to counter the stereotypes commonly held about midwives:

> Frequently, when only the *midwife* part of *nurse-midwife* is used or heard, a negative image is conjured up. This image is of the good-hearted, loving, but untrained midwife either of past history or in rural areas of the South today, or functioning as a birth attendant for those disenchanted with the present health care system. It leads to the irrational conclusion that nurse-midwives are an uneducated menace

representing a backwards step into illiteracy in the provision of mater-
nal-infant health care. (Varney 1987:29)

Independent Midwives

Independent midwives (also known as lay midwives, direct-entry midwives,
community midwives, and birth attendants) began to grow in number as part
of a countercultural movement in the 1970s (Arms 1975; Gaskin 1978; Rothman 1982; Edwards and Waldorf 1984; Reichman 1988; Sullivan and Weitz
1988; Susie 1988; Wertz and Wertz 1989). These midwives attended the
births of women who were disillusioned with the care hospitals were giving
women at birth and who wanted to give birth at home instead. These empirical
midwives learned in a variety of ways, including going to births and learning
firsthand, with no additional training. Some midwives apprenticed with general practitioners who still attended homebirths in rural areas, while others
apprenticed with homebirth midwives who were already practicing or at birth
centers run by midwives. A few even apprenticed with grand midwives. The
first schools for independent midwives were informal and based at midwifery
clinics where there was a high volume of births (including The Farm Midwifery Center in Summertown, Tennessee, the Santa Cruz Birth Center, and the
Maternity Center in El Paso). One of the first formal three-year programs was
offered by the Seattle Midwifery School, which opened in 1978.

This group of midwives is by far the most diverse in their education—
both in style and amount—than either grand or nurse-midwives. What unites
this group is where they attend birth—mostly at home or in birth centers.
The legal status of independent midwives varies from state to state; considered blatantly illegal in some states, in others it falls into a gray area depending on the definition and scope of practice, and in still others licensing is
required. In some states, such as Florida and Washington, independent midwives are part of the health care system and can receive both insurance and
Medicaid reimbursement.

Carol Sakala describes the unique care provided by independent
midwives:

> Formal studies and personal accounts reveal that women who work
> with independent midwives tend to receive from these caregivers, and
> deeply appreciate, care that is: individualized; gives the woman a pri-
> mary role in informed decision making; emphasizes health promotion
> and prevention; minimizes technological intervention and iatrogene-
> sis; addresses physical, psychological and social issues; and conveys

dignity and respect. Nonetheless these midwives may attend less than 2% of births in the U.S. and their impact as direct caregivers is relatively small. (Sakala 1988:1150).

Nancy Wainer Cohen's description of independent midwives consists of a list of what women who use them say:

> They are gentle. They don't injure their clients; they don't use medical interventions; they are so kind to your bottom!; they aren't on a power-trip and they don't make you feel guilty or inferior or inadequate; they are patient; they know the meaning of "support"; they don't think the doctor's word is God; they understand your fears; they are willing to talk about death, not skirt the issue; they are strong in a very loving way; they love babies!; they love women; they know how to listen; they are intuitive; they explain things; they are emotionally accessible; their hands are soft, firm, and welcoming; they let me cry and complain; they are warm and compassionate; they are knowledgeable and wise; they know how to build confidence; they're very special, every one of them. (Cohen 1991:163)

She goes on to say that midwives attend births rather than deliver babies and are not medically trained, seeing themselves as outside of the medical establishment. They do not try to separate themselves from those with whom they work by utilizing the symbols of professionalization (e.g., uniforms and formal hierarchical relationships), but are an integrated part of the community they serve.

Physician's descriptions of independent midwives provide another perspective. Some consider independent midwives unqualified, incompetent, irresponsible: an ACOG official statement accused these midwives of "maternal trauma" and "child abuse" ("ACOG Official" 1977). In a survey conducted by sociologists Deborah Sullivan and Rose Weitz, physicians voiced their views on the licensing of independent midwives in Arizona. The majority of the obstetricians (74 percent) and general practitioners (63 percent) wanted to outlaw homebirths attended by licensed lay midwives. Some felt that it was regressive to use midwives and stated: "Their patients die! Their babies die! It is Third World medicine." Another writes: "Arizona must protect its desired unborn from McDonald counter girls who subsidize their income delivering damaged babies" (Sullivan and Weitz 1988:136). The physicians expressed concern regarding the lack of standardized training and the limited nature of midwifery education. Sullivan found that midwives believe that physician opposition stems from concern about midwives' educa-

tion as well as assumptions that homebirth is unsafe, and they feel that doctors fear midwives' infringement on their practices. The survey of physician opinions supported these beliefs (Sullivan and Weitz 1988:141).

The major question that independent midwifery poses in the public's mind is the safety of homebirths, especially with midwives who have no standardized education or practice requirements. Research and primary attention in the medical literature have focused on safety. The ACOG came out with a statement in 1979 that homebirth is not a reasonable or safe choice; to support their opinion, they used statistics for all births that occurred outside the hospital, including unintentional and unattended births. Thus, premature births in malls and taxicabs and accidental homebirths with their high mortality rates were grouped with those homebirths that were planned and midwife-attended. Subsequent retrospective studies have shown that homebirths with trained attendants have significantly fewer mortalities than homebirths that were unattended (Burnett et al. 1980; Hinds, Bergeisen, and Allen 1985).

Lewis Mehl designed one of the few critical studies comparing the safety of homebirth to hospital birth for low-risk women. He matched 1,046 home- and hospital births and found no differences in deaths or neurological damage of babies. The attendants for these births, however, included both physicians and midwives, so no specific conclusion about the safety of independent midwifery could be reached (Mehl, Peterson, and Whitt 1977). A more recent study comparing the safety of home and hospital births evaluated the statistics from births attended by the midwives of The Farm in Tennessee. This study, like a number of others, suggests that "under certain circumstances, homebirths attended by lay midwives can be accomplished as safely as, and with less intervention than, physician-attended hospital deliveries" (Durand 1992). (For a comprehensive review of all available studies of midwife-attended home- and birth center births, and a comparison of midwifery outcomes with those of physicians attending low-risk women in hospitals, see Rooks 1997.)

The ethics of the medical response to homebirth were considered in another medical journal, which reported that since homebirths do not appear to significantly increase mortality, to deny access for backup medical care either prenatally or at births is unethical, because doing so only adds to the possible dangers (Hoff and Schneiderman 1985). This article was written in response to some physicians' and hospitals' decision to harass those choosing homebirths by denying them backup care. This issue continues to be a problem today, in some areas adding unnecessary risk to homebirth.

In response to criticism from nurse-midwives, physicians, and others about the lack of standards, accountability, and mechanisms for ensuring competence, MANA created the North American Registry of Midwives (NARM) to set up a national certification process for the certified professional midwife (CPM). This process, which came into use in 1994, honors multiple routes of entry into midwifery, including apprenticeship, direct-entry schools (the term *direct-entry* refers to educational routes into midwifery and means that the midwife did not have to pass through nursing to enter midwifery), and nurse-midwifery training. Certification requires validation of experience as a primary-care provider with all phases of perinatal care, validation by a midwifery mentor of competent acquisition of a long list of required skills, and passing a challenging day-long written exam and a hands-on skills assessment administered by a qualified evaluator. The NARM certification process was created by direct-entry midwives, for direct-entry midwives. It emphasizes out-of-hospital birth and continuity of care. Its standards are based on a nationwide survey of what 877 practicing midwives (one-third were CNMs) deemed to be essential entry-level skills. At present, approximately three hundred midwives have been certified as CPMs, and the NARM exam and/or certification process has been adopted as the standard for licensure of direct-entry midwives in a number of states and Canadian provinces. The existence and increasing popularity of this certification among independent midwives indicates the commitment many of them feel to high standards of care, verification of competence, and professionalization.

Listening to Midwives

Since the 1950s, nurse-midwives have had their own professional organization, the American College of Nurse-Midwives (ACNM). The ACNM established standards for midwifery programs and certified as nurse-midwives those nurses who underwent subsequent training in midwifery, but did not bring in other midwives. Independent midwives began to network in the late 1970s, but there was no formal communication between nurse-midwives and independent midwives until the two parallel but separate groups were called together in 1982 by Sister Angela Murdaugh, then president of the ACNM. Thus was the Midwives' Alliance of North America (MANA) born.

Midwives who had trained and worked—some as independent practitioners and others in roles comparable to that of obstetrical nurses—outside the United States, Canada, and Mexico added their perspective to MANA.

MANA also explicitly recognizes and includes the third strand of midwifery: the grand midwives, who had been practicing before 1965 and serving women in the South and in immigrant communities. Through the Sage Femme Award given to those midwives who served communities locked out of the health care system, MANA recognizes the unique contributions of traditional midwives as they link midwifery from the past to the current developments in midwifery. By honoring these women for their skills and many years of service, MANA encourages other midwives to learn from them.

At the first international conference of MANA (in Milwaukee in 1983), I was particularly struck by the fierce independence of the participants. These women were drawn together by a desire to share information and support for other midwives. As midwives, they had been working alone in their communities, isolated from each other (with the exception of a few places in which vital midwifery communities had developed, such as The Farm in Summertown, Tennessee, and the Santa Cruz Birth Center in California). But many were reluctant to join an organization that might impose on the birth process a structure and rules that imitate the medical model that these midwives firmly rejected.

The key issues MANA has tried to address encompass promoting the education of midwives, establishing communication between midwives, and protecting the midwife's legal right to practice. The challenge has been to use the midwifery model to create standards of practice and routes of education on which this diverse group could agree. From the start, the members of MANA have stood steadfastly by their beliefs that women should be able to choose where to give birth and with what caregiver, and that midwifery should be decriminalized. At the same time, much of the organization's direction has been toward supporting national midwifery certification, the objective being to make midwifery more accessible and desirable to women by making it "acceptable" to the medical community, which holds both political and ideological dominance in our society.

This does not mean that disagreements and differences among midwives have faded; instead, as the three strands become intertwined through MANA, the concerns of each group evoke great controversy and debate. Yet the boundaries that separate midwives are beginning to blur with shared concerns.

As a regional representative to MANA I have had both the responsibility and the pleasure of fostering communication among many different kinds of midwives. The first prerequisite for communication is listening, and I

realized that my circumstances provided me with a special opportunity to listen to many women who had chosen the path of midwifery. The literature on birth and midwifery includes a wealth of accounts of mothers' experiences of childbirth and a growing number of autobiographies of midwives, but nothing that traversed the full range of midwifery in the United States today. So I began to use my travels to MANA board meetings and conventions to meet with and interview midwives.

In these interviews of two grand midwives, eleven nurse-midwives and fourteen independent midwives, I have striven to capture the diversity of midwifery. These women come from all parts of the country and from very different ethnic, religious, educational, and ideological backgrounds. They care for women in pregnancy, labor, and birth in a wide range of settings and with significant differences in philosophy and style.

Some of the questions came from listening to midwives who have radically different concepts of midwifery or come from backgrounds different from mine. I wanted to know how midwifery affects their lives personally and how the stresses in their lives affect their midwifery. I asked if they think midwifery is a feminist issue. I asked them how they were drawn into midwifery, and how their personal birth experience affects their work and their perceptions of birth. I asked how faith or spirituality affects their practice, and how they deal with the fear that inevitably comes with difficult births. I wondered how other midwives deal with the stress of attending births in a society hostile to midwifery, especially independent midwifery.

In an introduction to her phenomenological research on women becoming mothers, Vangie Bergum comments on how research about others affects the self:

> Through the dialectic going back and forth among the various levels of questioning there is striving for a thoughtfulness, "a deeply reflective activity that involves the totality of our physical and mental being." In one sense, it is an exploration of self, forcing a self-reflective attitude. I have been forced to attend to the question of "Who am I?" as a woman and a mother. (Bergum 1989:14)

And I would add "as a midwife."

The interviews took the form of a conversation, with no formal structure. Even though I had prepared specific questions, the interviews were open-ended. I followed the conversation as it flowed and did not ask each of the midwives all of the questions. Some of the women knew just what they

wanted to talk about, so I went along. Others responded to the questions. This fluidity of format seemed as natural to me as the course of a birth.

The interviews took place at conferences, in the midwives' own homes, or in their offices. Whenever possible, my sister Sarah came with me and took photographs. I learned that the setting affected the tenor of the interview—some were conducted over breakfast before a long day of workshops, some in between board meetings, and one occurred when exhausted from a conference we both lay down on the hotel bed to talk. Just as in midwifery and prenatal care, we were interrupted by family and other pressing events, and children were often in and out. As midwives, however, we are used to reaching important, intimate places in a short time, just as we do in our work. As a result, the interviews often reached a depth of intimacy that facilitated profound self-revelation. I sat with women as they shared painful stories through tears. Such stories touched me, as did the tellers' willingness to be so open. The interviews were transcribed from audiotapes and then significantly reduced in the editing process. In the tradition of oral narrative, the voices come through as the spoken rather than the written word.

Even though none of my words are included in the oral narratives presented here, my questions frame the answers and my selections make me a co-creator in the story. This fully interactive and nonobjective relationship is analogous to the practice of midwifery. Just as each midwife chose what to say, I chose what to save and tell as that person's story.

Because I am a midwife, and in some situations an acquaintance or a friend, many stories were told to me in the casual manner that one midwife uses to talk to another. Certain expressions were used that other people might not understand, like certain birth lingo (e.g., VBAC). For the reader's convenience, I have tried to explain these in brackets within the context of the oral narratives.

The format used to present the midwives' stories follows the tradition established in *Our Bodies, Ourselves* (Boston Women's Health Book Collective 1979), in which individual stories are used to create a larger vision of women's issues. This tradition reflects my own path to midwifery. It was through the stories heard in women's support groups, and later from listening to midwives' birth tales, that I received my education about women's bodies and women's lives. I learned that by listening to individual stories, one can create a collage of more general truths about women—or in this case, about women as midwives.

At this point in the process I can see who is missing from these portraits.

I am missing the strong voices of foreign-trained midwives—those who have been trained and have worked in other countries before coming to the United States and have struggled to fit into our system, either as CNMs or as independent midwives. As my own vision begins to broaden to include midwives throughout the world, I miss their perspective here. Originally my intent was to interview midwives throughout North America, but I was ultimately unable to include Canadian or Mexican midwives. Their proximity to the United States and the fact that midwives in both countries hold membership in MANA ensures that developments in midwifery in these two countries will be closely connected to developments in the United States.

Canadian midwifery is at a particularly exciting point in its history, as in province after province direct-entry midwifery is becoming both legal and a fully integrated part of the health care system. In Mexico, traditional midwives still attend the births of more than half of the country's population, mostly in rural areas; nurse-midwives attend women in hospitals in the cities but are not allowed to catch babies, and a new breed of professional midwife who seeks to combine the best of both worlds is gradually emerging (Davis-Floyd, pers. comm. 1997).

Two other types of midwives that I was unable to interview are male midwives, of whom there are a few, and physicians who work as midwives (Ina May Gaskin calls these M.D.'s "midwives in disguise"). I also wanted to interview a midwife whose primary focus was conducting research. There are so many more stories to be told and recorded; this is only a start. For every midwife included, I wanted to interview five more. Just as there is no end to the flow of women's birth stories, so also there will be no end to the midwife's tale.

Presently standing on the periphery of the health care system, I support the struggles and achievements of nurse-midwives who work within the system. I honor their contribution to the group of women who feel safest with them and to whom they have greater access by working within the system. I also honor the grand midwife who works in her own community without access to, or belief in the need for, the particular level of technology that I, as an independent midwife, would feel uncomfortable working without. Even though I practice in ways very different from both, their wisdom and expertise in midwifery can only broaden and deepen mine—if I listen.

Midwives are as diverse and as similar as the women they serve. In spite of their differences, however, I see them all, in the words of MANA's theme song, as "sisters on a journey." I visited each of the women included here to

listen to and record her version of the larger story, to understand in some small way her personal reality of being a midwife. I extend to you now the invitation to listen as I did to the individual voices of these midwives and to look at the tapestry woven by their stories, noting both the harmonious patterns created by the common threads that link them and the tangled strands that indicate areas of conflict and disharmony.

Sisters on a Journey

Portraits of American Midwives

When the streams of talk we collected are gathered together,
many hard truths are revealed. But in addition, putting together
many individual voices has produced a resounding chorus. The
exhilaration and the wisdom in this chorus tell us of many
visions of life, different for different women and powerfully
different from the reality that now holds sway.

—Emily Martin
The Woman in the Body:
A Cultural Analysis of Reproduction

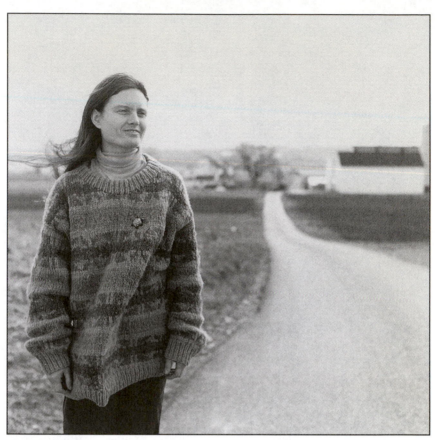

Rondi Anderson

Rondi Anderson is a nurse-midwife who serves primarily a large Old Order Amish population in Lancaster County, Pennsylvania. Nursing and midwifery students as well as family practice residents visit her practice to observe as part of their education. Rondi had a homebirth practice for ten years and worked for two years as a nurse on a Navajo reservation before she became a nurse-midwife in Utah. She is a member of the ACNM homebirth committee and of MANA. Rondi has published in the *Journal of Nurse-Midwifery* two articles on retrospective descriptive studies of homebirths attended by nurse-midwives, one based on statistics from two homebirth practices, and a recent one that examined homebirth practices nationally. The low infant mortality rate for the births in this study supports previous research that planned homebirths with qualified midwives can be a safe choice.

Rondi Anderson

Birth is important to women—that's why it is important to me. I spoke at a NOW [National Organization for Women] convention this fall, even though when they first brought the subject of birth to the state organization they said they didn't think it was a feminist issue. I think birth is missed by a lot of feminist organizations. I talked about how the medicalization of birth is very male-oriented and that women are not very respected by that system, even raped by that system, and nothing is being done about it both in terms of safety issue outcomes and psychological outcomes.

The first birth I went to was my own. I found it powerful and very amazing. I was in awe—it was like nothing I had ever done before, and it opened up a whole awareness of other possibilities for me. I think I was very much strengthened by it; I was only nineteen. Not that labor wasn't painful. I felt betrayed by Ina May Gaskin [author of *Spiritual Midwifery*] because she talked about how contractions were rushes and all you have to do is not be afraid and be in good shape. I was jogging right up until the ninth month of my pregnancy. I was totally counterculture; not one part of me thought I should be in a hospital. But contractions weren't "rushes." I didn't feel scared or that "there's something wrong here." I felt like, "You lied to me. This is not a rush. This is pain." I wish somebody had said that to me, that "this is going to hurt, and you're going to be able to do it. It's part of the process. There's pain in life. This is one of the times when you're going to have to deal with it."

It was the most pain I had ever felt in my whole life, though the birth to me was as ecstatic as the labor was painful. To me I felt like it was a cycle, an incredibly intensified life cycle. I liked it. I felt like the pain was as integral a part of it as the powerful ecstasy of the birth.

Anyway, I felt like the birth was so positive and so empowering and strengthening, and gave me so much. I went to a hospital nursery to visit a friend of mine's baby a month or two after my baby was born. I was just taken by these babies all in a room without their mothers. I couldn't imagine somebody taking my baby away and putting it far away from me in a nursery. I would kill them maybe, taking my baby. I felt like the hospital just didn't respect what that was for a woman, what birth was and how much of the incredible experience I had was lost to these women. To think that it was really okay to take their babies away and put them in nurseries. It just wasn't okay, as far as I was concerned. I wanted to let women know that they had alternatives and to help provide safe alternatives for them. I was driven—passionately driven. As much passion as I have ever had for anything. I would have done anything to be able to be involved with birth, to be able to fulfill my mission.

I found a lay midwife and a family practice doctor who were doing homebirths. First I started working with childbirth education. Then six months after my daughter's birth they started inviting me along on births. Within a year and a half after her birth, I was attending births alone. I did some home study and went to lay midwife conferences. I did quite a bit of reading and a fairly high volume of births.

I had done maybe a hundred homebirths before I ever went to a hospital birth. Going to a hospital I felt totally intimidated, and the medical community treated me like I was basically dirt. I wasn't even allowed into hospitals a lot of times. And I didn't have self-confidence; I didn't know what they were doing enough to be able to stand up to them. I think that there was a part of me that wasn't sure whether I was inadequate and that they didn't know more than me.

I also felt like I really couldn't reach people that had any kind of high risk because as a lay midwife I had to work with the cream of the crop. I thought that if I got more education that I would have more access to the more needy population. I also come from an academic family; both my parents are college professors. So I went to nursing school. Those years weren't particularly hard; I was just sort of playing the game. I didn't mind the mental stimulation and felt accepted enough there. It was in some ways good for my

self-esteem: "See, I can get A's. Now here I am the midwife that you think is so bad, and look it. I'm playing your game and can get A's." In some ways it made me feel kind of cocky. I had started practicing midwifery when I was twenty.

The hardest time for me was when I was working as a labor and delivery nurse. I hated how things were managed, and I didn't have control over it. I got frustrated with the people I was working with, and they got frustrated with me. I was a midwife, and even though they all knew that I had been a midwife, they still saw me as a nurse. I had a lot more knowledge and skill than what I could use, just because they didn't want my input. That was very hard on me, and I really had to sit on my hands a lot. The deciding factor of when it was time for me to go to midwifery school was that I made a male doctor cry, because I was so frustrated. It wasn't even that big of a deal; all he wanted to do was rupture somebody's membranes, and he wanted me to go in and set him up for it. I had seen two or three people have their membranes ruptured and have cord prolapses [a rare occurrence in which the umbilical cord comes out before the baby's head, shutting off the baby's oxygen supply and often leading to fetal death]. The mother was laboring fine; progress was good. There was no reason to do it. He just wanted to go in there and meddle, and I basically told him that. He felt so intimidated by me, and later I found out that he went to the back room and started crying. I thought, Well, I think it is time for me to go, move on.

I went to graduate school in Utah because I wanted to continue doing homebirths, but I didn't want to alienate the medical profession. I wanted to show them that this really was a viable alternative, and I felt like I needed the degrees for them to be able to listen to me. I basically just got tired of being an outlaw. I liked my master's degree program a lot, and midwifery school was good. Even though I had to play the game in midwifery school, it was much better than being a nurse. I got more experience in prenatal care and well-woman care too. It was kind of nice to watch other midwives, both as a nurse and as a student. I think there was a part of me that felt I had really gotten into midwifery too fast, too young at only twenty years old. My skills were good, and I was motivated enough so that I was fairly educated. I don't think I was really unsafe, but after the incredible responsibility of delivering babies, in some ways it was nice to just step back and watch other people do it and say, "Okay, teach me for a while."

I learned how to suture there, and I hadn't done that before. I rarely suture now, maybe every four months or so, but I do know how. My hand

skills [positioning and use of hands when delivering a baby] are okay, so I have a fair number of intact perineums [the area between the vulva and the anus; it stretches or tears when the baby is born], but even if they tear I don't usually suture. That's the nice thing about doing six-week exams postpartum. Often I can't tell which ones I've sutured and which ones I haven't. They all look the same. It's very rare that they don't heal up just fine.

After school I knew that I wanted to get back into homebirth, so I wrote to all the midwives who said that they were doing homebirths listed in a directory put out by the American College of Nurse-Midwives. I told them who I was and asked them if they needed any help. Most of them wrote back and said, "We would be glad for you to come to the area but there's not really a demand for another midwife in this community."

Penny [Armstrong] wrote back and said, "I'm thinking of leaving my practice. I would be very interested in having you come and take over." It just seemed like it had my name written on it, and I had to do it. Penny made it very easy for me. It just seemed perfect that I could go right into an existing practice working with Amish clients for whom homebirth was something that was a norm in their culture. I think that is one of the big challenges with homebirths right now. If you're working with the middle class, they're having to deal so much with their families and their friends and the medical community saying that it's unsafe. There's a lot of issues because of that.

Plus the Amish don't sue. I hope that never means that I give them less quality of care, but that is certainly an issue when you are doing homebirths. I carry malpractice insurance, but even if you carry malpractice insurance, who wants to be sued? I think that doing homebirths is really a setup to be sued, particularly if you're a professional. I never thought about it when I was a lay midwife, but when you're seen as a professional, if anything goes wrong and you transport to the hospital, and the medical doctors there say, "If you would have been in a hospital . . ." They talk from a position of authority, and people psychologically at that point need something to blame it on. It's really easy to get blamed, even if it is something that happens all the time in the hospital. It's just nice that I don't have to deal with that. Right now, nurse-midwives aren't getting sued that often, but doctors are—60 percent of obstetricians have been sued. People sue right now for all sorts of things. You almost have to look at your client as if they're out to get you or something, or deal with them as if they are. I don't have that mentality at all when I interact with people. Yet when you're doing the volume that I'm doing, you get all kinds of people.

About 80 percent of my midwifery practice is with the Amish. They are a wonderful population for me to work with. They don't have the implicit trust in the medical profession that the mainstream does. They feel safe with midwives and don't feel like they should be somewhere else. They're farmers. They're real earthy and give birth very unpretentiously. They're not flowery; it isn't like this big anxiety-laden event in their life that they have read about for years. Even though this is a generalization, they see birth as part of life, and I can relate to that—it's how I like to help women give birth. It is something that they know that they want to do and they just need somebody to help them do it.

They do tend to have fast labors. They're like the Navajo in a lot of ways. I've worked only with people that have unmedicated births, and in that they're all pretty similar. I've never worked with an epidural [regional anesthesia used to deaden the sensation of contractions during labor or for surgery] population, which is unusual for the United States, where epidural rates are very high.

With the Amish, most of the time you have a sense that you're dealing with someone from a different culture. I'm sort of oversensitive to it and tend to want to go out of my way to not stand out or offend people. The Amish do amazingly well with it, but I am struck by the images that the local non-Amish people have of Amish people. There is a real bigotry: "They're uneducated. They're dirty. They're unfriendly. They're cold."

A lot of that comes from people having interactions with them on the street, where the Amish will sometimes put out a very icy exterior. It comes from being treated like the monkey in the zoo by the tourists. Tourists will come this close [*gestures*] and photograph them without saying anything. It's gross what happens. I think people don't think about what that does to people. When my nursing students come with me to births they say, "Wow, I couldn't believe how friendly and intelligent they were, and their houses are so clean." I spend a lot of time just educating the students about other cultures. We're all really the same in a lot of ways. We are more similar than we are different.

I do really like working by myself, even though I don't feel one hundred percent good about it. Although I know all the clinical textbook stuff, I think I do work intuitively, a lot. I have trouble with anybody who has a dominant opinion pulling on me, expressing their perspective—it interferes with me feeling like I can focus on the labor and what needs to be done. Obviously if you get there and the kid is being born, it doesn't matter who's there. But if

I'm dealing with a labor where I'm having to make choices about management, it's hard for me if I don't have somebody that's closely connected with me, and I just don't have that person. Yet I do have a childbirth educator that I take to births with me sometimes, but she has to be very passive. Some of it is monetary though too. It costs more if you work with two people. The more tired I am the more I want to work alone. Some of it is I just don't want to be distracted in the middle of the night and have to deal with someone else's energy. I want to be able to just focus on the birth.

I realize that this is an issue for most people and that the American College of Nurse-Midwives includes in their statement on homebirths that you have to have two people there. I do bring the nursing students, but they're just observing as part of their OB [obstetrical] rotation. The schools want to get them to see advanced nurse clinicians—not that they're learning to be midwives, but to be exposed to one of the things that nurses can do. Some of them come for more than that.

One hard thing about midwifery is sleep deprivation, which I think is a constant challenge. Another is the incredible responsibility of holding life in your hands and having to look back and say, "If I had done it this way . . ." I haven't lost a baby yet, but there is always the potential of death. I sometimes feel just incredibly weighted down by it.

Also I hate dealing with a medical profession that isn't supportive of me. It makes me crazy. I can ignore it until I bump up against it, and I'm reminded of it. Our backup obstetricians tolerate us. They don't think that we're the most wonderful thing that ever happened to birth. I don't think that it is competition; I think it's that they really can't justify what they're doing, if what we're doing is okay—to have your babies at home. For the high-risk patients you can, but a lot of people that the OBs take care of are low-risk patients. Birth is such a loaded thing for people. All cultures have their rituals that they surround themselves with that make them feel safe. For an obstetrician those rituals are very hospital technology–oriented. They can't imagine that it's okay without the fetal monitor, without the IV [intravenous], without all that stuff that they have in the hospital. Therefore, what we're doing must not be safe. Even though they know the volume of births we do and how rarely we have problems. It's much more of an emotional thing than intellectual. Also, I think that obstetricians, particularly female obstetricians, tend to be harsh. I think that OB residencies are so very brutal, particularly on women. It's almost like being an abused child except that it happens to be when you're an adult. You just cannot

come through it without having been hardened. I think that surgeons are often the same way.

Another tough thing in midwifery is being on call. Although I do all right with it, I think that I don't realize how much it wears on me, not being able to take a schedule home. I also feel like my lifestyle is so different from everybody else's. People aren't on call all the time. People aren't up all the time. People aren't dealing with, and this is actually something I love, the kind of intimacy that's at birth. I feel like it sets me apart socially; it's hard for me to know the social cues that other people have since what I do is so different from what everybody else does. It's sometimes difficult to integrate back into the mainstream to get my social needs met. And part of it is that people don't get it. Sometimes I'm just incredibly exhausted. People just have no concept about what it means to have been up the past two nights and to have just dealt with this incredibly intense labor. They look at me like, "Well, what's the big deal?" Certainly, women who have been in labor are the most aware of what that might mean, or mothers who have children that stay up all night too.

Sometimes if I've done a million births and I'm so wiped out that I can't deal with people, I'll call up and cancel on people even though I'm not at a birth. But if I'm honest and just say, "No, I just can't do it," then I have people start rolling their eyes at me. They would rather I say that I'm at a birth. I find it's a great excuse; you can always use it.

I think that there is something very elemental about a laboring woman where personality is beside the point. I can usually walk into any labor and just tune in, just click right immediately with her and have it be okay. I know labor—not that people's labors aren't different, but there's just something about a woman in labor that allows that kind of intimacy to develop very quickly. That's one of the things that I want to do as a midwife is to let women have a relationship with me, where they can trust me, and I can be there for them when they're in labor, but I can't do it a hundred percent—I really do burn out so I take off every third weekend. If I don't do that I can really feel the difference and I get so that, when I get a labor call, I don't want to go. Or I'm sitting in her house with her and I don't want to be there. That's not fair to anybody either. Definitely, I have some guilt when I do go away for a weekend and miss births. Sometimes I know that if I had been there, it would have been a more positive experience. Not that I think that I'm wonderful, but I think that there is an important relationship between the midwife and the laboring woman which develops over time.

I'm glad for my lay midwifery experience, and I think that it was very valuable. I think that if you just go through the nurse-midwifery training you don't have the whole picture—not that I have the whole picture. I think that nurse-midwives can be kind of snooty toward lay midwives. I think that there's a lot of valuable knowledge base in lay midwifery that nurse-midwifery doesn't have. I think that the nursing component of nurse-midwifery means that midwives are biased toward the hospital management.

One of my problems with nurse-midwifery is that they don't do apprenticeship training. I think that apprenticeship training is very important; to start with observing and working with somebody that you trust, who wants to train you, and with whom you have a close relationship. And to not have to go into practice until you're really feeling comfortable. In nurse-midwifery you never watch; the first time you do it, you do it yourself with someone watching you. And that person is not necessarily on your side. It's a fairly impersonal relationship with your clinical faculty, which is sometimes even antagonistic. You go in and do it, and they watch you do it and critique how you did, which was okay for me, because I had delivered many babies at that point. But it wasn't okay for my fellow students; they were terrified. They didn't know what to do and were just doing everything that they could to do it the way that they knew that the instructors wanted them to do it, because if you do it wrong they yell at you and give you a bad grade. You're under so much pressure anyway in graduate school. It's not a nurturing connection between an experienced midwife and somebody that's learning. The students are supposed to have been all labor and delivery nurses who have watched birth, but nurses don't watch birth. They shoot the pit [pitocin] in, they run around and do the things that they have to do. They're not sitting there focusing on watching the delivery for the most part.

I don't think that student nurse-midwives will have the confidence at birth if they're really pushed into a situation before they're ready. Their clinical base is very small; you only have to do twenty births before you're done with school. Then you end up with clinicians that have some real insecurities about birth. Any time you have that fear, you end up having people that probably intervene more, probably don't have as much trust in the process or respect for the woman's intuitive feelings about giving birth. They probably feel like they need to be doing something all the time, which can be a weakness of nurse-midwifery.

One thing that I always see is that lay midwives really are the best with perineums [the area between the vulva and anus; it stretches or tears when

the baby is born]. Lay midwives don't focus on manipulating the baby as it comes; they focus on getting the baby's head over the perineum and then the baby just comes out—you just sort of receive it. Since my nurse-midwifery training I've changed how I do it, but I think that's probably typical. Once you have that image of that stuck shoulder behind the pubic bone, and what you're doing is bringing it down—it's very hard to just leave your hands off and let the baby come.

Doctors do episiotomies because they're sure that everyone is going to tear, so they can't find out that it often doesn't happen. Doctors are so insistent on having women be in a certain position when they give birth because they can't deal with how they are going to maneuver the baby if she's on hands and knees. When you're a lay midwife, it's not an issue, because you're not maneuvering the baby. You're dealing with how you are going to support the perineum.

Originally I learned that from watching. Maybe not everybody can learn that way, but my mentor didn't teach me a lot. She just midwifed, and I watched. I read. When I could figure out what was happening, I just did it. I stepped in when I could see that I was helpful.

I think that it would have been okay for there to be more of a formalized program, but there weren't any back then. I think that just the first step to learn this trade is to let me watch you as my teacher. That's what I do with my students, I make them watch me. The nursing students, even the residents, I make them watch me and then they can pick up what I do, take it and integrate it in their own stuff. That's got to be the first step. Maybe it's not for everybody, but it certainly was for me. I see that with lay midwives. I think that gives them a confidence about birth. You need to have confidence in the birth process in order to really be perceptive. When you're scared, you can't pay attention, because you're too wrapped up in your own insecurity. When you're feeling confident you can pay attention and focus on what you need to. I now have many nurse-midwifery students. I like the teaching part, and it's sort of my little mission that keeps me going, that I'm going to change the world. I mean every nurse that I take out, if she has a positive experience, is going to go to her workplace and say, "Homebirths and midwives are really okay." I think the more that I can reach people that way, the more I feel like I'm letting women know that they have safe alternatives.

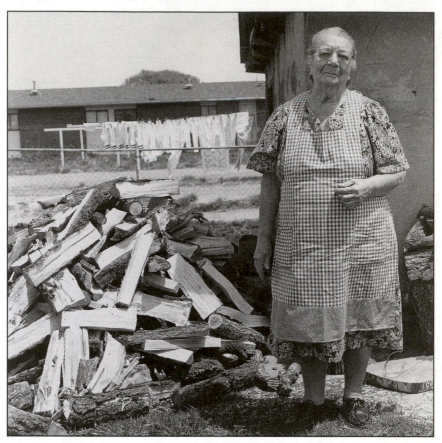

Jesusita Aragon

Jesusita Aragon is one of the last traditional Hispanic midwives licensed to practice in Las Vegas, New Mexico. She grew up in the mountains of northern New Mexico. Forced to leave home as a young woman due to two pregnancies out of wedlock, she struggled to raise her family alone, building her own house and running a small farm. She gradually became a well-respected midwife in her community and had women come to her house to give birth. In 1989 she was recognized for her years of work by receiving the Sage Femme Award from MANA. This interview was conducted primarily in Spanish, with the help of an interpreter.

Jesusita Aragon

I've been a midwife for too many years! I delivered my first baby when I was thirteen. My grandmother was a midwife, and even though I went to school, she taught me everything. She wasn't home when I had to deliver that [first] baby. But I remembered what to do. I already knew from when I was a really small child. My mother died from the flu when we were very young, so my grandmother took over raising me and my younger sisters. I am the only one still alive.

During the first birth I attended, my grandmother was forty miles away at another birth. I wasn't afraid. My grandmother told me that if you're going to be a midwife, you've got to keep your mouth shut. And so if you see the butt coming or you see the feet coming, you don't say a word and scare the mother. You just attend the birth and you keep your mouth shut.

They wouldn't let me go to school after eighth grade. Since I couldn't be a nurse, I decided to be a midwife. It always interested me, I always liked it. I wanted to do it. And I'm still a midwife. God gives it. I've never had any problems really with my health other than my eyes. I am eighty-five years old. I am healthy, no headaches, no stomachaches—thanks to God—no cramps, no nothing.

It doesn't make any difference being older; I am still as strong. I can still attend births. And when the day comes, then I'll say, "I can't do it." I do not feel tired. I can deal with being deaf, but I can't deal with being blind, so I ask

God not to take my vision away. The most important thing is *the feeling* of what you're doing—your hands feel everything.

Midwifery comes from the heart. This woman who came back to see me from New York says she never forgot me. Many years ago she showed up here in labor when I was with another woman in labor. When she showed up at the door she had no money, she was alone, her man had left her. But I never asked her, "Do you have money? Can you pay me?" After I was through with the other birth, I attended her birth and never asked her for any money. Then she left and went back to New York. Now her daughter has gone to college and she later found a man who is treating her well. They came back here because they never forgot me and how well I treated them. And they gave me a check to pay for that first birth!

I attended a birth fifteen years ago of some people from California, and every year since they have sent me a card at Christmas—only this year they didn't and I'm worried about why—maybe they were hurt in the earthquake or something.

I have babies everywhere. Once a woman was visiting from Germany and she wanted a midwife to take care of her. She came and found me to deliver her baby. They were still in the United States, in San Francisco, when the baby was one year old, and they sent me a card saying, "Today, my baby is one year old. . . . thinking of you." And then she went back to Germany and I haven't heard from them since. I hope someday they'll send me something.

At a birth I feel very happy and hope that everything goes well. If there is a problem, I'll bring them to the hospital. The woman who is in that photograph there had a baby—and she had a very hard birth. I helped her and she helped, too. If the woman doesn't help, it doesn't happen. It can be a hard birth and it will just keep going and going and going . . . but if the woman doesn't want it, it won't happen. I was going to take this woman to the hospital because the baby was so big. And she said no, she wasn't going to go to the hospital—that she wanted to deliver it with me. She said she would help as well. They would both do it together. So, we did it together and God helped us. The baby was almost thirteen pounds. *Muy grande.*

My grandmother said that for forty days after a woman had given birth she could only have an egg with onion and toast for breakfast. For lunch she could only have chicken or the meat of a male sheep, not a female sheep. For dinner only a gruel made out of wheat or corn or oats. But I don't believe in

that. Women don't have that diet now. Now, after two or three days, they go right into the car and out to dances!

Not that many women breastfeed, but they are starting to more now. If you nurse the baby, then they don't get sick. They don't get diarrhea. If they get a bottle, they get sick, they get diarrhea. But with nursing, they don't. I tell them not to stay in bed. They shouldn't do work or exercise, but they should walk around. Before the women were much stronger—they were happy when they were going to have a baby. And now the women aren't as strong and when they are pregnant they say, "Oh, I don't want to have this baby." But if they get pregnant, they have it anyway.

I listen to the baby with my hands. I am in a videotape showing how to turn a baby. You can do it if the woman hasn't started labor; if she's started labor, you can't do it anymore. You go looking for where the head is—and little by little turn it.

Women must go to the doctor when they are pregnant—to have blood tests and so the doctor can say whether they can have their babies at home or not. They make sure everything is okay, with the baby's head turned down and everything like that.

I had a good relationship with the doctors. Sometimes I would have women come, and they would say, "Oh, I don't want to have my baby here, I want to go to the hospital, I want to have a doctor." I would call Dr. Haverston or Dr. Clark and they would come over and reassure the mother that everything was fine. "You can call me if you need me, but everything's okay." The doctors trusted me. But I don't know about the doctors now—I don't work with them.

When I went to a birth at the hospital—and when the doctors would let me deliver the baby—the nurse would say, "You have to put on gloves." But the doctor would say, "No, she doesn't have to, she works with her hands."

I examined a woman once who felt like she had a tumor, so I sent her to the doctor. They operated and then the doctors called and had me come and look at the tumor they had taken out of the woman. The doctors believe in me.

There was a woman who was seven months pregnant and her uterus was ready to fall out of her. The doctors told her they would have to do a cesarean to get the baby out and also remove the uterus because it had prolapsed so badly. But the woman didn't want to do that, so she came to me and asked me if I could cure it. So I moved the baby up and moved the uterus up and fastened the uterus with a sash. The uterus never came down any more and the baby was eventually born without any problems.

When it seems like the uterus is going to come out when the baby comes out, and you can see it coming down, you should grab it with a clean white rag and hold onto it and move it back. Don't let go of it. Even when the placenta is coming, don't let go. Afterward, put a sash on and tighten it so the uterus can't come down.

The longest labor I have seen is thirty-six hours. It was that long because she didn't want to push. There are births that just come slowly. The woman may have a contraction every hour or every half hour. But it's okay— it's just the way that it is, and it's fine that it's slow. I'll be making tortillas, or talk with my friends, and the woman can be in here resting a little bit or talking to her relatives if she brought them—whatever she wants to do.

If the baby is born not breathing, I suck the mucus out with a bulb syringe and then I pump air in. Then I pick the baby up by the feet and hit it on the bottom. There are some babies that are born almost as if they were drowned. Sometimes I massage the heart gently and sometimes it works, sometimes not. If it doesn't work, the baby dies. It is nobody's fault. It is just what happens.

I pray at births, but nobody knows what I pray. And everything is okay, thanks to God. I never lost a woman. Oh, some babies, you know. Some of them born dead or died a little while later. You know that. It's not your fault. God always helps me. I pray when I take care of a woman. The baby sometimes dies.

One time a doctor delivered a baby in Taos about fourteen years ago. There was a suit against the doctor and so the doctor came to me asking me to come and give a word in support of him. He wanted me to testify in the court case. And I said, "Why me? I don't have the education." And he said, "Yes, but you have the experience." So I went and I testified. When I got there everybody [in the courtroom] knew me because I had delivered so many babies for all the people there! We won the case. The same woman was pregnant again when I went there. The same lady. She went to the hospital and the baby was born dead—the second one. After a baby dies, I spend time with the mother afterward. I stay with her a little while and counsel her and tell her that these things just happen. Sometimes they just have to happen.

The most difficult skill for a midwife is knowing whether it is a false delivery. If somebody comes and they are having labor pains, it may not be that they are going to have their baby then. Maybe it will be later on.

Sometimes people don't treat you well. But you have to treat them well. When they come, you have to be nice and make them feel comfortable.

The chamber of commerce is going to give me an award on the first of May. I have lots of awards from the city, from the governor. I have delivered 45,927 babies—twenty-seven sets of twins and two sets of triplets. Too many babies! I used to deliver 200 or more in a year. Every day, every night, every moment. I used to work at the parachute factory and my boss let me out to deliver babies. He was a good boss. I worked eleven years over there. I never sleep! A midwife never sleeps! As soon as I get into my blankets to go to bed . . . "Jesusita, we need you!" You never sleep. Isn't that right? If you want to be a good midwife and treat people good, that's the way you have to do it. Smile when you're coming. And oh . . . treat them good. So they can feel better. But the most rewarding part of being a midwife is that I am appreciated by the people.

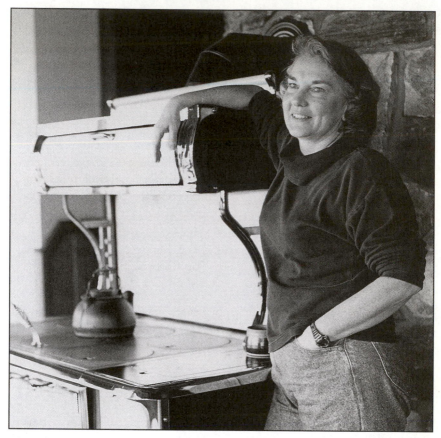

Penny Armstrong

Penny Armstrong, CNM, was born in Maine, where she worked as a health planner and a social worker helping problem teenagers before becoming a midwife. She went to midwifery school in Scotland and then took a refresher course at Booth Maternity Center in Philadelphia to practice in the United States. Penny has worked in a number of nurse-midwifery practices and had a homebirth practice for ten years in Lancaster County, Pennsylvania, primarily serving the Amish community. She then worked in Cooperstown, New York, where the midwifery practice included serving high-risk women in the hospital. Penny has coauthored two books with Sheryl Feldman, *A Midwife's Story* and *A Wise Birth,* as well as writing a number of journal articles. She continues to live in rural Lancaster County, Pennsylvania, and has served as the clinical director of the Community-based Nurse-Midwifery Education Program (CNEP), which offers an at-a-distance midwifery training program.

Penny Armstrong

People fantasize about writing books, and a lot of midwives think that they have the ultimate collection of birth stories, and even though they want to do it, they just can't because of all the constraints of work and publishing. I never would have undertaken writing a book in a million years. It was just totally foreign to what I was doing, and what I was interested in. It's fun to be able to say what you want to say and have it make a little tiny bit of difference somehow, but it's not why I was born. I wasn't born to do this, like I was born to swim, or like I was born to midwife, whereas my friend Sheryl was born to write. She eats, drinks, sleeps writing. It's her entire existence. Her dream has always been to be a writer. So once she had raised her two teen-aged sons, she came here to stay and write the great American novel. To make a little money she worked for me at my prenatal clinic, answering the phones and that sort of stuff, and she started following me out on births. Then she left and got a job as a governess and was traveling around Europe working on the great American novel. She said that the stuff that happened here just kept coming back to her. What she had seen here at births with the Amish kept surfacing, and she couldn't get the novel stuff going. Finally, she decided that she would just come back and write *A Midwife's Story* just to get it out of the way so that she could write the great American novel. After she had finished *A Midwife's Story* she was going to just put it away, and a couple of her friends said, "Well, you know, you should do something with it." I

said, "You definitely don't want to do anything with it," because she had written about a lot of things that only a best friend knows.

Sheryl and I had been best friends for thirteen years through multiple husbands and all sorts of other stuff, and that was all in there. Fortunately, the editors in New York did not want the real personal stuff. They just said, "It's not appropriate—take that out." Thank you, the first three chapters of my life are gone. It was easy—I covered up a whole marriage and everything.

After it was finished, I didn't really want it to be published because I didn't think the Amish community would appreciate it very much. So we had a big crisis about it, because she was my best friend, and this was her lifelong dream, and she was on the verge of having it realized, and it was in direct conflict with everything I basically believed in. I decided to give up. My brother gave me really good advice. He said, "Penny, (a) nobody's ever going to buy it and (b) if somebody buys it, nobody's ever going to read it. So don't worry about it." The only time that my brother's ever been wrong in his entire life.

So Sheryl decided to just give it a try and had it published. A nurse-midwife said to me, "We're really glad that there is finally a book written by a nurse-midwife; too bad it has to be about homebirth." Within my profession it was met, except for a couple of my friends, with a resounding silence. It's interesting, because that was six or seven years ago and now it's mainstream. We jokingly call *A Midwife's Story* "The Little Book That Could," because it just sort of keeps chugging along. Everybody's sort of picking it up now and reading it and saying, "That's a great story."

One agreement that I made with my publisher was that there wouldn't be any publicity here in Lancaster County for the book, so I thought that maybe nobody would ever notice. I was so paranoid and didn't want to violate the trust of the Amish whose birth stories we wrote. I was just waiting for the wrath of the bishops to come down on my head, or be put on the blacklist. I even thought that if they publish this book it would be the end of my practice.

After scrambling the stories to try to protect everyone's privacy, my Amish friends felt that I didn't end up telling the truth. Even though I tried to explain to them, they don't feel that there was any explanation for not telling the truth. They don't understand poetic license. And then they loved to tease Sheryl about one mistake that she had made—that there wasn't shoofly pie at a wedding because they wouldn't serve shoofly at a wedding. She still insists that there was at this wedding.

The Amish may be the only intact birthing culture we have left where there is a community of people that truly believe in birth. They have an unbroken chain of birthing; not ever knowing twilight sleep or forcep births. They don't know pitocin from anything, they don't know any other way to birth, they don't watch TV, and their friends don't know any differently either, so they have a real cultural imperative to birth, they have the expectation that they will do it. Most other women today, you have to try to empower them to birth.

People are often puzzled about what the Amish do. It doesn't seem logical to have diesels to drive their milking machines when they won't have a television set. Their decisions are all based on what they absolutely need to have to keep the family unit intact, and access to safe birthing care is one of those things. They'll show great forgiveness if people run them over in their cars, shoot them, or if they rape their women they'll go to court and say, "We forgive them, and ask that the court give them leniency." And yet they'll fight if you take their midwife away.

I like to tell stories, and the Amish love to hear them. Nine-tenths of my work is story-telling, and the Amish have a great sense of humor. We'd sit at the kitchen table while the mom is contracting and we'd talk, and the kids are gone and the husband is there and we tell stories.

This one woman told me, "We can sit here and talk and laugh and we can do cherries and stuff, but when I throw up that's when the baby is coming." The Amish always seem to know—you come in and they say the baby is going to be here in an hour, and you know they are right. So we are sitting there laughing and doing cherries and she gets up and reaches for a bucket and starts throwing up, and she gestures, and I look down and there is the baby's head between her legs. And as soon as she stops throwing up she says, "I told you so." I had no idea that she meant *right* then.

They love stories like that, they love birthing stories. You can tell birthing stories generic enough so that they don't know who it is. They also like stories from the outside. I had a student who was working with me who lived in a highrise in New York City. And they just loved to hear New York City stories.

The experience that I had from working with the Amish showed me that the farther you get away from the earth, the farther you take birth away. I think that each layer, each hospital floor takes you farther away from the earth, then you lose the connections to the rhythms and the cycles. You can't reproduce that in a plastic environment.

About a year and a half after *A Midwife's Story*, Sheryl came over one night and said, "I think we ought to write another book." I said, "I don't want to write another book." Sheryl's very wily, very political. So she gets a bottle of wine and we're sitting drinking wine by the heat of the stove. She says to me, "So what would you like to write about?" Big mistake, she had a tape recorder hidden. I remember the night, because I was really hyped, and I was pacing back and forth. So she taped it and then about three weeks later she came over one day and plumped down the outline for *A Wise Birth*, and she said, "Well, how about this?"

So we co-wrote that book. We really had a lot of trouble with the two voices because we have really different styles. We got an advance for it, but when we took the first draft of *A Wise Birth* down they threw it in the wastebasket and said, "This isn't what we wanted. This isn't what we paid you for. You can either pay us back, or you can write what we want you to write."

That was my worst nightmare. So fortunately, shortly after that our editor had a baby. She was a thirty-nine-year-old primipara [woman having her first baby] when she had a baby with a nurse-midwife. The next day she pulled *A Wise Birth* out of the wastebasket. People in New York are very New York–centered, and if you don't deal with the issues the way that New York people are dealing with them, then they don't exist. It's really powerful, especially for publishing. They wanted us to talk about a New York issue—the effect of sex discrimination in the workplace on women who are pregnant, and the effects of rape on women, and just a lot of stuff that we weren't talking about. They kept saying that they wanted us to toughen it up, not make it so soft. It was a long, painful process.

Actually, we have one more book that both of us want to write. The first one *Sheryl* wanted to write, the second one, *I* really wanted to write. This one we *both* want to write, and no one wants to hear what we have to say. We want to talk about poor women having babies.

Writing *A Wise Birth* tired me out, even more than I already was. It also taught me more about birth history than I ever wished to know. We read every book that had ever been written on birth. I've got them all upstairs in crates, and the mice are going to eat them before I ever open them again. If you write a book and put all this work into it—blood, sweat, and tears— when it comes right down to it, you will not believe the things that you're willing to compromise in order to get it published.

I had this little pact with myself that if I ever got a call in the night, and there wasn't really a compelling reason to go, but my instinct told me to go,

and I couldn't make myself go, then I would be finished with midwifery. And that happened, and the next morning I said, "That's it, I've got to stop." I just didn't have it anymore, but it was real subtle. I didn't want to stick around like a broken-down athlete, and keep doing this after my time was finished. I know that the reason I was able to have the kinds of outcomes that I had over the years was because I minded my shop really closely, and I didn't cut corners. I just didn't want to fall in that category. I also had this flash that something might happen. I mean I always considered my work here blessed, and we, the birthing women and I and their families, got away with an incredible amount of things. We were sometimes teetering on the edge between bad and good outcomes, and they always tipped to the good. I thought one of the reasons for that was because they have a direct line to God, but you also have to give yourself up to their way—which may not make sense or match your way.

So, there was a sense in me that it was time not to do births anymore, and I didn't have a real rash reason for not doing it, so I just kind of let it evolve. I didn't fight it. It just changed. It wasn't like all of a sudden I was fearful of birth, but I just had this sense that it was time to be done, and that I was pushing it, every day that I did it thereafter. I was very careful, and I just tightened my ship, because I realized also that I lost maybe a little bit of the edge of my instincts, so I tightened my ship, extra careful that I made sure everything was done properly. I very carefully picked the person that was going to be my last birth, which was someone I had worked with five times before, and she was low, low, low risk. It was going to be a fun party, and I went out and, of course, she had a cord prolapse [a rare occurrence in which the umbilical cord comes out before the baby's head, shutting off the baby's oxygen supply and often leading to fetal death]. "Do I really want to do this? Haven't I just done this? Haven't I done this enough? Excuse me. Can I please be excused?"

Another nurse-midwife moved here and made it even more possible, because she could just step right into my practice, and I didn't have to worry that my clients were okay. I thought that it was really important for me to get out of the kitchen, and kind of leave the cooks to stew their own pot. It was surprisingly easy for me to say that someone else is here, and they're safe. That's all I really cared about, was that they had options, and that they were safe, and that was taken care of. I didn't feel compelled to be sticking my nose in and doing that sort of thing, but it's very hard for people to understand that they couldn't come up to the house or call me, or that I didn't want to

hear all the complications that I wasn't going to solve. I basically functioned a lot like a general practitioner. Not so much in a medical sense, because I was pretty careful about that, just kind of a jack-of-all-trades. We went to people's homes, and we saw that the grandmother needed this and that, and we arranged those things. So, I was really a primary caregiver, in a pretty pure sense of the word. That was a hard part for people to give up, seeing me as a primary caregiver. So, I thought I better get out of the kitchen.

My husband and I went up to Maine to a camp we have up on the Canadian border, and we stayed up there for a year and a half. We had a great time, and detoxed. It was great. I had a couple of friends that said that within six months you're going to think that you've peeled off all the layers of your exhaustion, and you're really down to the core, but you aren't. It's going to take a lot longer than you think. I think it's sort of like grief in a way, it moves in stages.

At first I was real energetic. Oh boy, sleeping at night! Then all of a sudden I realized I was tired to my core. If something would wake me up at night, I would cry, because I thought I had to get out of bed. And a lot of things came up that I had put away and hadn't dealt with for ten years. Life was really on hold, because my practice took priority over everything else. It had to be dealt with. I didn't even think about anything else. I sort of thought, "Well, maybe my life is over? I'll just enjoy doing art and stuff like that. I don't have anything else left in me as far as careers or creativity." I was perfectly willing to let that be the case.

I remember thinking that I was dead, spiritually, that the part of me that just rebounds—which is an important part of my being—was gone. Not to overemphasize the negative part of it, but very few people are honest about the cost of this kind of work. No one wants to hear about it either. Everybody wants you to be a hero. They want you to be what they need you to be, which is one of the problems that I have. People have taken it really personally that I am tired. I've actually had people get angry with me because I'm tired.

Now, in the profession it's a little bit better. It used to be that Sister Angela [Murdaugh] would stand up at our ACNM convention every year and say, "Midwifery is a mission. If you're not on a mission, get out," and everybody used to stand up and cheer. A couple years ago she stood up and said it, and about half the people in the room booed. I think there's a real change in attitude. It used to be, "Give all you got and then give some more, and if you can't do that for some reason, then you are less than a midwife," but I think that mentality is changing somewhat. More people are going into it with

families. It used to be that single women, nuns, and people that didn't get married were nurses. In fact, when my mother-in-law was a nurse, there was a rule in the hospital that she worked in that you couldn't be married. She secretly got married and kept on working. Now that there are older women becoming nurse-midwives and nurses, I think all that's changing.

I think it really helped me to have one person in my life say, "Some day you're going to be an older nurse-midwife who will retire, you're going to be too tired to do this, and that's going to be okay." That was the sort of phrase that I clung to. Whereas I think that ten years ago, there was so much opposition to our practice of midwifery that we didn't know if they were going to be strong enough to wipe us out entirely or whether we were going to be able to survive. Now that there's a little more security, there is a little bit more room for people to question what they are doing and maybe move in and out of full-time practice. If you had a job in nurse-midwifery ten years ago and left it, nine times out of ten you couldn't get another one. There just weren't any jobs. Now there are about three jobs for every nurse-midwife. That has really changed the call to midwifery.

About a year and a half after going to Maine, I came back and by that time I was healed enough to start to ask questions again, to wonder about stuff, to visit Kitty Ernst [a CNM who has been active in the promotion of birth centers and in community-based nurse-midwifery education] and talk to the students she was working with in her midwifery program. One of the students came up to me afterward and said, "You have to be my preceptor." I said, "I can't do midwifery anymore." She said, "No, I'm serious. You have to be my preceptor," and about two weeks later the hospital where she was going to go called me up and said, "Do you want to come and do a short-term stint and precept a student?" I love to teach, so I thought, "Oh, why not, maybe I'll find out some things. Maybe I'll find out how much of what I believe in translates to the hospital."

So, I went up there and precepted her for three months and got back into the practice of midwifery. I stayed up there for about six months, and now I do it intermittently. One day I called the office to say, "I'm having this problem with this student, what should I do?" and they said, "Gee, I don't know. Don't ask us. You figure it out." When I talked to Kitty one time, I said, "Gee, Kitty, we need to be doing something about clinical supervision. We need to have some resources for the preceptors. The students need a little bit more intensive advisorships." So she said I should work on that.

So I eventually returned to develop a formalized preceptor training pro-

gram for midwifery instructors. I basically teach midwives how to teach clinical skills—especially how to demystify and put words to the art of midwifery. Many of our most valuable midwifery preceptors were saying, "Well, that's just the way it is. I don't know how I did that—it's just energy. I can't teach these students. I don't know what I do—I just do it. I can't break it down." And the poor student is standing there going, "I'll never understand this. I don't have whatever magic it is that she's got. I'll never be a midwife." And they get really discouraged.

We developed this workshop to teach people how to demystify their practice and also how to handle student preceptor problems. We taught about adult learning, how to diagnose learning style differences, and understanding what it's like to work with a forty-year-old woman with three children who wants to be a nurse-midwife. She brings a lifetime of experience to her work, and that's different from dealing with a traditional student, maybe a bit younger, with less life experience. So we started that workshop, which we do on a rotating basis throughout the United States.

A lot of the students from CNEP are people from birth centers, and they already have practices, they are already serving their communities, or they're from religious groups. Or women whose husbands are lobster fishermen who can't leave the coast of Maine because they can't fish anywhere else. They've been sitting there, dying to be nurse-midwives for ten or fifteen years. It is just giving a way for those people to get their certification in midwifery.

I don't know about the future of midwifery. I don't know what is holding women back from using midwives except that I think there is a cultural imperative to separate women from birthing, to separate families. I think there is a cultural imperative to separate us from the earth from which we get all of our powers and from our animal instincts. And I think that that movement is much more potentially dangerous for us as practicing midwives than all the laws of any state or country. How do we stop this disintegration, this taking apart of our birthing culture? We have thousands of years of weaving together this rich birth legacy, and since the turn of the century in this country we have absolutely ripped it apart. We have silenced women, anesthetized them, tied them up, doped them to the max, and now we expect these same women to rise up and say, "I want midwives? I want to take back my power?"

It isn't going to work that way, so we need to work with one woman at a time. The only change we are ever going to see has to come up from the ranks of mothers and babies. And what is going on out there with our society,

with our politics, and with our families that is preventing those women from standing up and taking charge of their own health care, their own maternity, and their own birthing? What kind of societal pressures? As midwives we cannot make a difference; the change has got to come from women themselves. What we can do is be out there giving excellent care to mothers and babies. And that politicizes women. How many female lawyers had their first baby with a nurse-midwife and then became really politically active? That's how Tipper Gore got started. She had her baby in Nashville with a nurse-midwife and now the word *nurse-midwife* is sacred in the Gore household—which is helpful because their house happens to be one of those in Washington that can have some influence.

Even with the dream of having ten thousand midwives by the year 2000—that is just going to equal the burnout rate of those of us who are dropping off the other side of the world. Because how can you go in there and practice nurse-midwifery at the rate that some of us practice it for more than ten years? If anybody can, the more power to them. But when I got to be forty-five, the old bones didn't want to creak out of the bed. So I'm looking at the potential students that are coming—if you are twenty-five or younger, I love you, if you are fifty and want this dream, go for it. But if you are twenty-five I'm going to invest my energy in you, because you are going to replace me.

I'm not sure what is going to happen to us as midwives, especially when I hear there is this kind of midwife and that kind, and this kind of exam and that one. I would just like to say there are multiple pathways to becoming a midwife, with the end result being that we give safe, satisfying, culturally sensitive, and professional care. I need to know that the mother's and baby's needs are met.

I was able to participate in health care reform because of my activities in rural health care. I remember watching the early days of health care reform and listening to the speeches and thinking that this is one thing that I would really like to participate in. I am a dinky nurse-midwife in rural Lancaster, Pennsylvania. I am not a political person, yet about a month later the phone rang and it was one of the reform people asking me to participate in the process. I thought this is an unbelievably different way from how the previous administration worked, to be called up and asked what I thought should be done for reforming health care for mothers and babies. So I got my suit on and my briefcase and went down to Little Rock and sat at a table with Joycelyn Elders and others to discuss what maternity care was going to look like

under national health care reform. I heard them speak proactively about woman-centered birth and woman-centered health care. And whether we ever see those dreams realized, I know that there are people in incredibly high places in Washington who know the word *midwife*. For years we have been going around and saying, "Excuse me, I'm a midwife," and people would say, "What is that? What do you do? You must carry around a satchel and have dirt under your fingernails?" So there is some change and there is a little hope, with more awareness than before.

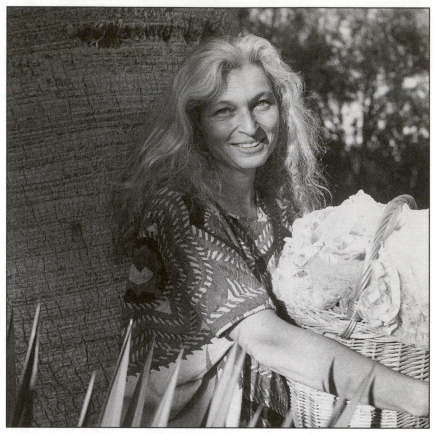

Jeannine Parvati Baker

Jeannine Parvati Baker is a midwife who advocates "free-birth" and runs a correspondence course for midwives called Hygeia College. She and her husband, Rico, have six children, five of whom were born at home, including a set of twins and a breech birth. Jeannine's last births were water births attended by her husband, and, from this experience and others, she supports couples who want to birth by themselves and works with them in prenatal and postpartum counseling. She has been a prolific author; her works include *Prenatal Yoga, Conscious Conception, Hygeia: A Woman's Herbal,* and numerous articles for psychology and midwifery journals. She is a midwifery teacher in the shamanic tradition and leads vision quests in the Utah wilderness. She is also an international speaker, archetypal psychologist, herbalist, and yogini. She has been nominated to *International Women's Who's Who* for contributions to medicine.

Jeannine Parvati Baker

In my life I sensed that there was something deep in me that was crying out for healing, that there was some original wound upon which all my other issues in life are based. Through that I had an inspiration one day to help others to remember their births, that I could work both ends of the continuum here simultaneously. I could be a midwife and help babies be born gently, as well as help the mothers and fathers remember their births, too, so they would be able to birth gently. I wouldn't have to do only reparative work, helping people who'd been damaged by their births, if I was also attending births and educating men and women about the importance of the baby and fetus's sensitivity to life, and to do the best that they can to honor the baby as a human conscious being. So that's how I got into midwifery, because I was wounded myself at birth. By exploring that wound deeply, as Hygieia, the Greek goddess of healing told me, the wound reveals the cure. So I looked at my own wound and came out through the other side into service.

That was before my children were born or even conceived, even before it became popular to break the "cycle of abuse," but I could sense in myself that I had a level of violence that would be perpetuated upon my children if I didn't attend to that. I was in a psychology program at a university. Previous to therapy I thought I wouldn't have any children at all. I couldn't see any need the earth had for more children. I was completely involved in zero-population-growth ideologies, plus I was also hurting too much myself to partake in the ecstacy of childbirth. I didn't even know that as a possibility.

To me it looked like pregnancy would be a burden, and taking care of a child would allow multiple opportunities for me to encounter my own violence. So I just said no to babies, and I was on my way through academia to obtain a Ph.D. Then after primal therapy I came to my embodied soul and felt that along with the maiden inside of me, there was emerging a new archetype—and that was the mother. And, yes, I would like to have babies. It took me only a year or two to convince my husband to have babies.

I have no training as a midwife. I have "untraining" around birth. I have divested myself of the dominating culture's ideas of what birth is. So I don't train myself, and I subsequently do not train others to be birth attendants. I say that I apprenticed to birth directly, and I will tell you how that happened. I am a yogini, I practice yoga. So when I had my first baby, looking back, that was what facilitated, along with primal therapy, my ability to be relaxed and alert, supple and strong, and to stay in balance and in my power. I ascribe that to yoga. By understanding *pranayama* (breath control), I was also able to assist my birth by breathing the way that felt appropriate at the time. So I wanted to share that with my sisters. I started something called prenatal yoga, and then I wrote a book. As I was teaching my prenatal yoga classes, the women would say to me, "I like the sound of your voice"; "When I'm around you I feel peaceful"; "I remember when I'm with you that this is my baby. I don't have to let other people take the experience." So I was invited to go to births. I went to many, many births. You might say I was a birth junkie, because I was so addicted to birth I'd drop anything that was going on, any time, any place, and go with the woman freely and sit with her in birth. I only came in the capacity of someone who was going to stay with her and breathe alongside. That was my whole role and job.

So I observed a whole variety of doctors. This was 1969 and the early 1970s, before I had most of my babies. I saw a lot of what I wouldn't want to do to help a woman have her baby, and much of what I thought were brilliant ways to assist a woman to give spontaneous birth. I saw a variety of practitioners in hospital settings and then eventually in homebirth settings, too. The next step was that women started saying to me, "My doctor or midwife won't help me because I've had a cesarean" or "because it's breech."

By that time I'd become a childbirth educator as well as giving birth to a breech baby and twins, so I was getting a little bit of experience under my belt. I decided since I had given birth and been through breech and twins that there wasn't anything to fear about this. Matter of fact, I thought they were easy births. Twins—double the endorphins, correct? I was ecstatic—

they were painless births. And a breech baby, from the mother's point of view, is a wonderful way of giving birth—seems just as natural to me as head first, or, as our culture is fond of saying, normally. I don't like to use the word *normal* at all, because it's from a Greek word that comes from the mathematical tool for measuring and I don't want to put some kind of a straight angle on my mind when it comes to giving birth.

I have birthed two of my babies in water and assisted others with water births, and I think it's a wonderful experience. One of the concerns was about, for example, the dangerousness of being in a bath with fecal matter when the baby's being born. I started perceiving that when you're in water, birth is so much obviously more sexual. You're in the same humor as sexuality—water. I saw it as disguising the same old "sex is dirty," saying, "That's the reason I don't do water births, because of fecal contamination." I just heard Dr. Michael Odent at the last International Symposium of Circumcision give this brilliant talk as a bacteriologist about the importance of inoculating the baby with the mother's culture, her inner culture, and that helps the baby's health for the rest of its life. So that was the last argument that likely held any water against this new phenomenon of giving birth in water. One of the best contributions is that it allows the woman access to her deep pleasure of birth, which may be a little tricky to realize when you have the pressure of air around you during the birth, gravity as a force working with you. So I highly endorse water births, and I encourage midwives to see how easy their work will be when they attend water births.

I'm very attentive to language, and probably one of my biggest contributions is the invitation to look at our language, especially the original meaning of the words we use. For example, in Hygeia College, I teach with an etymological dictionary. You can be precise with words to assist the woman in her own self-talk, so that she will be able to give birth with clarity in her unique way. Each midwife attends to her own language, because in the beginning was the word, and the word was flesh, and to help the woman have an authentic and original source experience is what birth is. Most of my ways of being in midwifery are through word medicine—or language you might call it—having an intimate dialogue with an intimate sister. And that empowers her to remember, This is my baby, and my baby and I are partners in this.

I just sort of take it for granted that birth is a natural rite of passage. It was an amazing discovery to realize that it was a spiritual passage as well. Having practiced yoga I had the template already formed—I was already

involved in a practice of self-realization through breath. Once I got into birth, undergoing that transformation from being my breath and having my consciousness and the baby's consciousness come together as one, I was ecstatic, which in the Greek means "opening from a small space to a larger one." It was an ecstatic experience for me, my first baby. And also it was an extremely sexual experience for me, an experience I had in amplifying degrees with each subsequent birth.

From the second and third babies what I learned the most was that nobody knows more about my body than I do. I began hemorrhaging during one of my labors. I went to the hospital. I brought my herbs with me, so I stanched my own blood flow with that, but I was concerned that I had a marginally placed placenta because of the volume and color of the blood flow and so forth. The blood stopped when I started to push, but then those guys got me in the hospital and said they needed to x-ray me, that my hips were a touch too small for these two babies about to come through, and started talking cesarean. I overheard them, and I left the x-ray department. They couldn't find me. They had never seen a woman in transition get up off the x-ray table and walk back to her room. I started packing to leave. What I learned is that regardless of where I am, I'll always be in power. Hospital, home, anyplace, because I did sign myself out and go home.

And I learned to trust my intuition, because both babies were born very ecstatically at home, and afterward I started another blood flow. The doctor followed me home from the hospital—he got extremely worried. I said to him, "I'll stop bleeding. You don't have to worry about this." I didn't receive any pitocin, nothing that would stop my blood flow. I just drank a cup of tea made from two herbs: shepherd's purse and bayberry bark. The doctor said, "Well, Mother Nature was in touch with you before, I guess she is again." I said, "She always is, because I am Mother Nature." That's something else I learned. We're not set apart from nature. The etymology of that word is related to the same word for birth. I was born, I give birth, I am Mother Nature.

My fourth, fifth, and sixth babies brought me to the present level of my work, which is called freebirth. In those births I didn't have to hire anybody, didn't have to pay anybody to be a midwife. I also didn't need any support, and this is kind of a new level. I consider it an evolutionary leap. It may be part of my megalomania to think it's so important. It's part of my vision for a mother to know that indeed if she's capable of conceiving a baby without the experts, she can birth one without the experts, too.

My role as a midwife has shifted into education through my word medicine and largely through my books, my articles. I am a member of the Association for Pre- and Perinatal Psychology, and through this new international friendship circle, my ideas are going out all over the world. So I have a public conversation going on about freebirth. I have been watching the freebirth community and have reconstructed all the arguments against freebirth—what people's concerns are about unattended birth. My vision now is that every mother, everyone, can be with her own woman as mother. It was this that brought me back a huge piece of my soul, and because of that I have a feeling of wholeness. I wanted to make that available to those who have the ears to hear. I'm not proselytizing or telling people what they should be doing. I'm confessing what I do, what I have experienced. I have many testimonials from people who have heard a tape of mine, read a book or article of mine, who have been inspired, because it reminded them of something they'd always wanted to do but had forgotten. There is a very large community of people having babies who go into birth without perceiving it as a medical emergency, but rather seeing it as an intimate sexual experience between lovers. Birth is a gentle emergence of the love that they experience with one another.

I do see the importance of healing the genders and inviting men back into birth. I notice there are many midwives now who also agree that birth is not only a women's mystery, but it's important to allow a man to be present. Our sisters know that giving birth is ecstatic. Even if we're in denial, part of us understands we're the Goddess when we give birth, so we enjoy that. I think also for very important reasons from an evolutionary point of view, we're hominids. I think we have a primal fear around men getting involved in birth, based on very ancient memories, or parts of our cellular consciousness have arranged it so that women and babies are protected when they give birth. The way I look at this is that every baby is from a mother and a father genetically in every cell of their body. The mother and father are pretty much balanced and represented in all of us. To have that show up at birth gives us cellular resonance. It lets us know that our inner experience matches our outer experience, at which point we feel home.

The great gift of religion is to tie us back to our souls. I think a lot of our religious quest is for us to regain what could have been a genetic retention of us knowing deep inside that we are loved. Our mother and father are both here as lovers to receive us, and that's what God is, that's what our source is, that's what divine parents are—our mother and father able to re-

spond to their original loving of us that brought us earthside. And to have other people around during the birth in supportive roles can in some way distract the intense bonding that occurs between mother, father, and baby, which I now call in my own set of scriptures "the holy trinity."

I confess I was for a time "in recovery," you might say, when I stopped attending births because birth was such a direct conduit to ecstasy. I just wanted to be in that energy field so much. But it came to me after I birthed my fourth baby that I had to start looking at how I could have ecstasy in my life other than attending births. There are many experiences in life that bring me that same feeling of unity that I have when I attend as a midwife, so I've gradually weaned myself from attending births in embodied form [meaning actually attending births]. I do attend births through people's imagination, because they say that they see me, or that something I have said has come to them at a really important moment in their births, and that I'm there as a guide for them. In other words, I've inspired them. I keep reminding them it's *their* imagination.

Plus I pray very strongly when someone calls me at the beginning of labor. I collect my family and we light a candle together to focus, and we say a prayer for the baby and let the candle burn until the baby is born. That candle that we see throughout that day or the next few days reminds us that a friend of ours is giving birth and we send to her our love.

Maiutic is a Greek word which means "in the manner of the midwife," and it is a philosophical term that comes from Socrates' tradition. In the Socratic model of education, the assumption is we have all knowledge already within and so, in the "maiutic way," the educator draws out innate knowing. I apply that directly to how I am with a woman in an intimate dialogue. I assume that if the woman conceived the baby without my help, she can birth that baby without my help, so I'm there to remind her of that, to return her mind back to that natural moment when she can give birth. If she allows the baby to signal and communicate baby's needs in the birthing process, she has all the guidance she needs. So a lot of our work is about clearing the road to birth, removing the "mind swaddling," that has been placed upon us by our dominator culture, the wraps on our consciousness that we have been given that estrange a woman from knowing from deep within to trust her intuition. And also, to communicate with a very conscious being who has the deepest vested interest in being born. That baby wants to come out. The baby incarnates because it wants to be born. And what the mother does is to look deeply at all of the obstacles she can throw off and remove the cultural stories

that do not support her in giving spontaneous birth. Also, depending on the woman, you may go pretty deeply into her own psychology, what occurred for her prenatally and pregestation and around birth, so that she doesn't have to reconstellate that experience. She can give her baby the best possible start by healing her own wounds.

Mostly I do it through talking and dreaming. You see, when a pregnant woman shares with me her dreams, I have a window into her soul. You get all of the psyche visible through the images of the situations of a dream, where the woman is at this moment in time in relation to her pregnancy.

I'm very careful, however, not to interpret dreams for pregnant women, just as I don't interpret a woman's birth experience, don't judge, assess, monitor, and definitely don't "manage" births. I'm not a birth enforcer. I'm willing to let the woman have her experience as it is. So I'm a very unusual midwife in the sense that I say straight out to a woman, "I have no medical skills. I don't know how to save lives. That's not my function. I'm with you as a woman. All I'm bringing to you is my experience. I've only delivered six babies."

That gets them right there, because they fantasize, oh my gosh, a midwife since the early 1970s, I must have thousands of birth experiences where I've delivered babies. "No, I've only delivered six babies, my children, because you are going to birth your own baby. I don't carry forceps, I don't do cesarean. There's no way I can deliver your baby. You birth your own baby. I have attended countless births, but I don't deliver your baby." And any time she's trying to throw me her power, I don't pick it up. I have too much of my own, frankly, to deal with it. I don't need to be in any way rescuing another woman.

Another profound lesson for women giving birth is in that great fear that we have about birth. We have a fear of pain, a fear of death, and also a fear of loss of control, too, that can correlate to those other two fears. Although when I look at the fear of pain, I see that it is still by and large a culturally induced fear. I know this from studying psychology and anthropology—if you are raised in a tribe that doesn't believe that birth hurts, then it's less likely that you will have an excruciating ordeal of birth. And then in our culture, where we expect birth to be painful, we also now have Hillary Clinton guaranteeing everyone's right to an epidural [regional anesthesia used to deaden the sensation of contractions during labor or for surgery]. I think that may be where subsequent drug abuse comes as the baby is being imprinted, following the mother's example because the mother and baby are so en-

meshed in pregnancy and even postpartum. They are in one energy field. So if the mother is taking drugs to deal with the fear and pain of birth and feeling out of control, then the baby internalizes this. Later, when their psyche is undergoing transformation in adolescence, they too turn to drugs, as their mothers did when carrying them.

So it's fear of dying, I think, that is really bothering women, because pain is a messenger that something's wrong in the body. So to have a fear of death comes with the territory of giving birth. As a matter of fact, if a woman says, "I have no fear of birth," I get suspicious that she is in denial, because I consider it quite natural to have some fear about an unknown experience, especially one that opens up the door to such a great transformation. As a mother, you shift to attending to another person's needs, and it's a big shift for someone to make.

The ego also dies or dissolves when you give birth. You move to a whole other level of consciousness. It's not just the "I" personally doing it, all myself, alone. You recognize that this baby is participating in the birth, and in my language I say that the Goddess is coming through me in birth, in this transpersonal experience. That is why ecstacy flows through me and during birth I connect with every woman who has ever given birth and ever will. At that moment when I have a baby emerging through me—I know we're two beings, but we look like we're one. It's a profound spiritual experience.

It is really important to meet a woman on her own ground so, if she's afraid of death, I say, "Well, of course." And then I invite her to journey with me into that. And we take what in shamanism is called a journey into the underworld, where we get to meet the great Inanna, who lives within that woman's soul. Inanna is important for midwives to understand, because she is the only one of the ancient goddesses who is able to go into the underworld and then emerge unscathed—a perfect model for the birth experience.

I teach others how to do this largely by confession, not by prescription, because I honestly don't know the best way for any other woman to be in her pregnancy and to give birth. Again and again, we drive home this point: no one knows better what's going on in a woman's body than that woman herself. And if she's in denial about it, we help her with it so that she remembers that she does have access down to the bone level about who she is. And no one else can tell her who she is.

I say, "Labor starts at conception," because I want to get off this bell-shaped curve idea of what birth is. As a construct it is very confining to me and has not been my experience as a midwife—that women always follow this

specific length of time between stages. Disconnect from the clock and get into a timeless dimension, because that is when you most clearly hear your baby's desires, how your baby wants you to move, even to breathe and shift your posture for this baby's birth. I think it's a good lesson for mothers, too, to surrender all personal desires to the baby's. If we do surrender during labor, then we may be more compelled to do it throughout the time that we are blessed to care for these babies.

From a larger perspective, I think all women are already mothers in the sense that each of us gestate with the eggs of our future children. While we are still inside our mother's wombs, we are all really mothers ourselves, because we have our eggs. So from my experience with dream states and altered consciousness, I've seen my children before they arrive. I've always had my babies with me. They've always been underneath my heart, carried in my belly, in my eggs. So this is a kind of timeless knowing of myself in capacity as mother, in intimate relationship with my babies. And then pregnancy and birth are a process of "womanifesting" to the world what my love looks like—in the form of a baby, but it already *is* me—in truth I am already a mother. When I gestated my four daughters I was already a grandmother, because their eggs were forming inside of me, their future children.

The first time I suggested to my husband that I wanted to birth with just the two of us present, he was totally freaked out. "No way, just the two of us!" He had too much fear. And he started hitting all of the obstetrical books I have all over the house. I watched him with mounting horror as he turned page after page, his face whitening all the more. I said, "Stop reading that! You're just scaring yourself with that." So he picked up midwifery books, and I can't say it was that much better. Eventually I came to invite him to attend our birth not as my doctor, not as my midwife, just as my lover. He said, "Yeah, I can do that!" So that's how we birthed our babies, as an erotic (which for us is a central, spiritual) experience—together.

And since I've had that experience and know how wonderful it can be, I invite mothers and fathers to reframe birth as the orgasmic result of nine months of foreplay of pregnancy. I tell them that it can be extremely pleasurable, as well as possibly painful. I encourage them to move through all of their experiences and not to separate themselves from what is going on. If they can stay with what is occurring, they will arrive at an ecstatic moment.

I learned a lot about giving birth from spending time in the wilderness. I say that's where my office is. Partly because it reminds me who's on top of the food chain. It's not me; it's not two-legged. We've got cougar in our

canyon. I'm allowed to step onto the wheel of life, and see that it is not a hierarchy with me at the pinnacle. Then I can connect more with the animal body wisdom that I carry in me, which is that spontaneous energy that brings forth renewal. I've observed out in the wilderness it's a rare buck that you see in a phone booth calling the vet to come and help his doe give birth because there is a complication. Wild animals spontaneously know how to give birth. It's domesticated animals, especially those that have been bred, such as chihuahuas and poodles, that have trouble giving birth and sometimes need cesareans. So to give birth naturally we learn from nature how to *be nature itself,* and then birth is really no big deal, no ordeal, that our minds can make it into. Rather, it becomes a natural consequence of heterosexuality.

One of my favorite slogans is that any child born in a hospital has experienced child sexual abuse. I take it from very subtle forms to the more obvious ones in stories that labor and delivery nurses tell where some doctors probe up a newborn girl's vagina when they're doing a newborn exam. I call that sexual abuse—to be touched by someone looking for what's wrong. And then of course circumcision, all the boys who have been mutilated by that ancient tribal cultural . . . It's a sadistic ritual! I was going to edit myself from saying that, but it is sadistic to circumcise a boy. He is a victim of child sexual abuse. The men are now coming on to that, finally. The men are now taking it up as their own movement to do something about that. And for the woman herself—I think any time I have not invited someone to come and touch my genitals, that's a form of abuse.

I know I'm one of those very rare midwives who doesn't say all births are painful. I know they're not. I've had three of my own babies without pain. I even have a video to demonstrate that birth is not an excruciating ordeal. I've also had three babies with some pain, but I can still have ecstasy with pain.

When you start licensing midwives you put a leash around your neck. What I have observed with not all, but many, of my sister midwives who were originally called to birth as direct-entry midwives, that when they went to get to their licenses, according to their state rules, they would learn a whole other medical way that really changed them, deeply changed them. There are very few midwives who can come out of that with the same trust that they used to have at birth, once they have been through the medical training, the program. And then, because you have invested all this time and all this money in getting a license, then you want to protect this license. And even if it's extremely subtle or unconscious, when you can have a license so that you can

practice more visibly or get third-party reimbursement, or whatever your motive may be for attaining it, then when you have to make some decision, when push comes to shove, you have to go the conservative route and stay within whatever standard or protocol your local board or state committee might have made. And by this you may do a disservice to the family who is giving birth. And this is their one birth. This is the baby's only birth this lifetime.

When you create licensing, you also create a legal and a right way to do it. And that law is going to classify *me* as illegal. If we all just totally give it up and say, "Get the state out of our bedroom," and we don't give jurisdiction over our sexuality to the government, then we're all in it together again. I also choose to live in Utah, which is a state in which parents can choose with whom they give birth. Pregnancy is not classified on their books as a medical condition, and neither is birth, thank goodness.

That's why I discourage midwives from putting that leash around the neck that by their own selfish concerns might yank them away from truly serving birth. It's not that I'm ragging on being selfish. It's really important that we know that we are midwives because we are being selfish. I am involved in midwifery for selfish motives. It's because I want more babies born on this planet who are deeply loved and bonded to their source, who are gentle beings, who are healthy, so that my children will be able to find suitable mates and I can have healthy grandchildren and then the earth can sustain itself. Because unless we bring in more babies that are able to be in resonance with the earth and feel connected to life, our planet is not long going to allow two-leggeds to continue our existence here. So, you see I have a pretty big picture of how healing birth is going to heal our earth. It is a selfish mode: it's not altruism that has drawn me to this.

We don't have to wait another generation to reclaim birth. I think it is an evolutionary step to have the men present as a lover between the mother's legs, so that the baby imprints on mother–father energy as partners. There's a lot of talk about partnership culture and how that's going to save the world. If you can imprint every baby that their being is mother and father who are in love, who are partners together, from the first moment earthside, I think you can bring about a partnership culture more readily.

I am open to being hired for consultations, and I do a lot of giveaway, too, when someone calls. I do charge for my time, and I get top wages from women who can afford to and feel prompted to pay me more. I have a really wide-ranging sliding scale. I've been paid anywhere from, well, you know, a basket of flowers and some beaded jewelry, all the way up to eight hundred

dollars I got for one session with a woman once because her CD happened to roll over. That was the day she got her interest, and she gave it to me because she valued it. I let the women give me what they value, because it's a value relationship. That's the important thing. It's between two souls here. I'm involved in midwifery still for soul-making, for my own reclamation of who I am, too. It's not only that I'm some kind of completed, finished being. I'm in the process of being all of who I can be, too, and that is through the relationship I have with the women giving birth.

If you can be self-sufficient at birth, maybe you can be self-sufficient after birth, rather than think you have to enroll in the cult of the experts the rest of your life to help fix you or because you distrust your natural processes, because you distrust life essentially. And that's a lesson we imprint on every baby, because we hire people to be around them just in case.

When I conceive my baby, I have only my husband between my legs. I don't have my midwife or doctor there just in case he might have a heart attack. Some men have gone into coronary conditions in the process of making love. But still, we haven't legislated men to be with experts just in case, have we? No, because we trust life, we trust love. For me, that's what birth is an expression of. It's bringing forth our love and showing it to the world. It's not this medical emergency that it has been made to be out of women scaring ourselves from our own sexual and primal energies.

Any kind of ceremony during pregnancy is an opportunity for women to bring more consciousness to their subsequent births. A Blessingway is the one that seems to be the most popular among midwives, though I really encourage communities to create their own based on their own soul. It's not only individuals that have soul, it's a community soul as well. Blessingway and Monsterway, are, actually Navajo rituals and ceremonies. I'm not Navajo. My father's people are from the Colville Indian tribe. I haven't been trained as that, so the ritual we have is more eclectic, but the backbone does come from the Navajo tradition. And that is to honor the mother and the father for bringing a new member to the tribe. It's a ceremony that's akin to a baby shower.

But as a midwife I attend the ceremony seeing it as another one of the fractals of birth, just as conception was, so I watch closely how the woman receives the gifts that come into her lap during the Blessingway, because for me it's a model for how she will receive the gifts of birth force energy, commonly called labor contractions or labor pains. Then I have a way that in subsequent time together or in conversation I may counsel her, tell her what

I saw, always prefacing what I say by telling a woman, "This is what I see. This is my fantasy about you, my experience. This isn't who you are. This is just what I am observing. What do you make of it? What do you think?" We'll have a conversation about it. It will often assist a woman so that she can settle into receiving the gifts coming to her lap in labor. I observe how she breathes, her posture, the other what you call portentous symbols that may come from who shows up and who presents gifts first, how her mate is with her during the ceremony, and so forth. From that we may learn new ways to clear the way for her birth.

Some feel that a Blessingway is supposed to be an all-women ceremony. Personally, when I have my babies, I have two ceremonies. I'm a Gemini. I like to have my women's community Blessingway and I like to have a Blessingway with my mate and all the dear men in my life as well. That's why I'm not a traditional midwife. I don't have a tradition, per se. Even my father's people who do have traditions, they've lost theirs. My dad was only five years on the reservation before he was shipped off into white man's world. Being an American, that gives me the freedom to choose what works best in the moment for us. Out of that we co-create new rituals that do serve us as we change and become more fully who we are.

I know from being an ecoactivist you must have biodiversity to sustain life. You must have babies born in all different styles, from the gamut of a huge party all the way down to the intimacy of a mother–baby birth. I wouldn't want necessarily for everybody to birth in my way, but I do appreciate that you're giving voice in your book to this perspective, because it's not often given much press. It's considered dangerous to suggest to parents that if they can conceive a baby without a cult of experts involved, they can birth that baby, too.

I would just ask midwives who have other belief systems to let us be. Let us have our experience without creating propaganda or finding ways to perhaps even snuff us out. I call that move "identifying with the oppressor"— when women who haven't had much power for very long start to get a little bit of it, they start to act like the ones who oppressed them previously. I have experienced this in midwifery groups that, because they think I'm dangerous to their perception of midwifery and to the cause that they're working for, work against what I am doing. I would just ask to be left to say my piece, too, and realize that this is supposedly a free country where each of us is to follow our own hearts in our work. I don't think you have to make somebody else or their practice wrong. I think you can have disagreements and learn from one

another without trying to suppress their work. That's what I would ask my sister midwives.

Heidegger's definition of the word *truth* is "let be," and so the truth for me in birth is to let be the family's experience. Actually, that's my highest compliment from a birth I've been at, when a family forgets I've been there. It's fully their experience and I have cloaked my energy so much to serve them in ways that haven't distracted them from their bonding. Then I think I've done a really good job as a midwife.

To co-create a world where we can remember we *are* nature, and live in harmony and balance *with* nature, and know that each of us is responsible for our own self—that is the imprint of a freebirth.

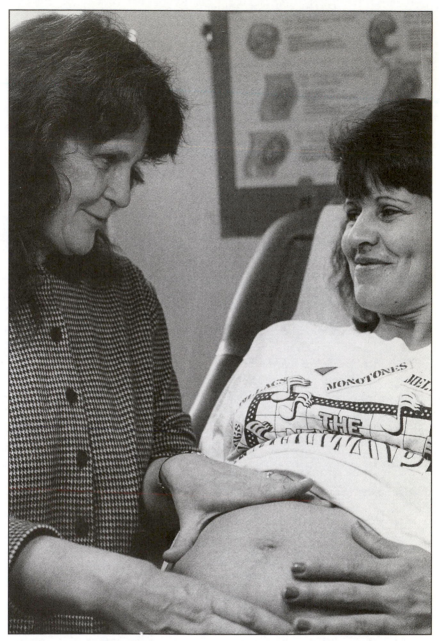

Connie Breece

Connie Breece graduated from the Yale Nurse-Midwifery Program and is a nurse-midwife with the Cambridge Hospital midwives. She has a special interest in international health and adolescent pregnancy. She is currently working at the Cambridge Birth Center, the first out-of-hospital birth center in Boston.

Connie Breece

I view myself as an organizer, and that spreads into all parts of my life, whether I'm teaching, being a midwife, working with women's health groups, going to demonstrations, or being with my friends and neighbors. I think of myself as somebody who helps other people move things forward. I always have. Before my midwifery training I worked in public education and literacy work.

When I was working in the seventies, I directed an education project in a women's prison. There was no prenatal education in the prison at the time, so we brought in nurses and childbirth education instructors to run prenatal courses, as well as GED courses, women's health courses, and English as a second language courses. In the late seventies, I was director of a school for court-involved young women who had dropped out of or been expelled from school. Some were violent, very troubled in every way imaginable, and many of them were pregnant.

That was my first big exposure to teenage pregnancy and young mothers. Later I chose midwifery as my work because I saw it as a concrete way to help. I saw medical training as dehumanizing to the people I knew going through it. I knew that I wanted to be a midwife and that I wanted to be able to work internationally. During nursing school I was angered by the demeaning treatment I received as a nursing student and by the treatment I saw trained nurses receiving. Watching the relationships between nurses and doctors was an eye-opener to me.

While I was at Yale, I walked into North Central Bronx Labor and Delivery for my training and saw these twenty-four midwives running the show. I was in heaven! And I learned from these very strong midwives; as preceptors, they were really good teachers. Then I did my integration [clinical midwifery placement] at Boston City Hospital. And I admit it: I really did become absorbed in the drama of the place. It's phenomenal when you're standing in a place where you can see *everything* in the course of a twenty-four-hour period—you can see life, and you can see death, and you can see drama, and you can see miracles. You can see everything there, and I was really attracted to inner-city work. Before I went to Boston City Hospital, I had met several of the doctors who worked there, and they were very supportive of me going there, and would say things like, "If you can be there for a couple of years, you really will learn not to be afraid of most things that you see." And they were absolutely right about that. It really did teach me that there's this wide spectrum on the wheel. I saw a lot of first-trimester and second-trimester abortions, premature deliveries—a lot of really sad stuff—pregnancies complicated by drug use, and a lot of beautiful deliveries, and a lot of complications.

Then, the midwives went through a really painful period at Boston City Hospital. Our service was growing at a good rate; we were doing nearly one-half of the deliveries there during some months. The problem was, we grew too fast for the physicians who were in control of policy about patient care. Midwifery philosophy, which holds that a woman in labor is essentially normal, and medical philosophy, which holds that anything can go wrong in labor, really clashed in those months. Arguments about women being able to eat and drink in labor, getting up and walking to the bathroom during a pitocin [a synthetic hormone that induces or enhances labor contractions] induction, the midwives' ability to care for women having a vaginal birth after cesarean or for women with asthma all took on grave proportions, and the tensions mounted daily. All trust between the midwifery service and the medical service disappeared, and the power to practice as we had been trained and as we believed best for the laboring women disappeared. It was a pretty excruciating decision for us to close the service the next May when we all resigned. It was an awful time.

You know, I see it as a disturbing trend when nurse-midwives become more interventive than they used to be. They are not practicing the way that we talked about when we first became midwives. Some of the practice settings in which we work, it's very easy to pick up those tools and games and

props and use them, especially when we're in difficult settings, with complicated labors. I have a lot of hope for midwifery as a whole moving forward together though.

What has to happen to get delivery, to get birth back to the midwifery model? I believe that the philosophy of midwifery really comes from that concept of guardianship. You guard the woman's spirit while she births, you guard the baby's spirit while it's birthing, you guard the labor spirit, and once the baby is out of the mother, you guard the baby's spirit—all of that. It takes a tremendous amount of energy in these times, when a lot of the people we come in contact with don't have the concept of spirit, or forgot about it if they ever did have it.

I feel very privileged to work with the women I work with. One of the reasons I love practicing at Cambridge Hospital is being able to provide care for the Guatemalan and the Salvadoran women. It is a phenomenal experience, because they are not out of touch with what birth is. You know, they come from a place where birth is very normal. Women have their babies at home, and they have their babies with midwives.

The years that I worked at Boston City were really rich for me because we took care of a lot of women from Africa and different cultures where birthing is still very much a powerful thing in the life of the family. It's not something that's been absorbed into medical structures or been taken away by a group of other people, of professionals. It's very pure and clean in that way.

And on the other hand, we also take care of a lot of women from Brazil, where in some parts 80 percent of them have cesarean sections! I just was with this woman in January. I wrote a note next to her name in the log: "She is the first woman in her family to try to deliver naturally. She has four sisters; there are fourteen grandchildren, and her mother and her husband's mother, and all the sisters, and every one of her siblings have had cesareans."

So when she was in labor for seventeen hours and was in a lot of pain and was losing it, she was having a real hard time keeping faith that her body knew what it was doing. She had this textbook labor: perfect dilatation, perfect course of progression, everything was perfect. In the last seven hours, there were at least ten other family members in the room begging me to take her to the operating room, take her out of her pain, give her a cesarean section. What was wrong with me? I was so exhausted by all of them and I couldn't believe it. So I just kept saying over and over again, "There's no reason to do a cesarean; this woman's body knows how to give birth. Just

don't lose your faith." You should have seen the birth—it was unbelievable. When the baby's head came out, the three sisters were here next to me, I had both mothers behind me, and cousins on the side—just a circle of faces around when the head came out! Every single one of them was weeping uncontrollably. They had never seen a birth before! The birthing mother had never seen a birth before. It was incredible! I just wanted to go to Brazil and say, "Stop this madness." They're making millions of bucks off all the cesareans, and they're in control of the birthing process in that country, and a whole culture of women believe that they can't give birth to their babies.

It's hard for midwives to organize, but we do need to make sure that a certain number of us take time off from our practices and do organizing. I could see not attending births for a year and just doing full-time organizing on behalf of birth and midwifery at some point. I'm not there yet; I don't want to do that right now, but I could see that in the future. And giving ourselves the social permission to do that, as colleagues, and as friends, and as sister midwives, is a pretty crucial thing.

I usually think of myself as a planetarian. I don't think of myself as being from a particular country. I think of myself as someone who's living on the earth, and that there are universal forces that guide us all along, and we're in a place in the universe that's gotten pretty out of touch with that. I think part of the work is to move people back toward what those forces are. And there are few places in daily life where you get to watch them at work as much as you do at a birth. So I do feel very spirited when I'm at a birth. And I really feel that as soon as the baby's head comes out, my work just takes on this whole other perspective; my job then is to see that the baby gets what the baby needs. And whether that's turning the lights off and shielding the baby from the light, or making sure the baby gets up on its mother's skin, or waiting to cut the cord . . . there are a million things that go into that period. In a hospital setting it can be as exhausting as the labor to protect that baby's needs at that point, but I feel really committed to that. I'm willing to wear myself out about that, as much as I am about all the other stuff. That's why I love homebirths so much, you don't have that.

I went to see this psychic last year who did a soul reading for me. And she told me that these years are good years in my work, in my life's work, that it's very important, that I'm supposed to deal with the transitions in people's lives, because I'm a good guide through transitions. She didn't even know that I was a midwife; I didn't tell her. And she said, "You are around a lot of babies, and birth, and stuff right now, I can feel that energy about you; that's

really important." But she said, "Your main life's work is you're going to help people get over to the other side." I said, "You mean death work and not birth work?" And she said, "This is preparation work: watching people go through transformations in this part of your work is giving you a base for what your work is going to be at the end of your life." So we'll see; who knows? Life is long.

I have worked for the past three years in a prenatal clinic here in Boston where we provide care for women from El Salvador and Guatemala and have been moved to tears not only by the hardships and pain in their lives but also by the strength with which they keep pushing forward. I have learned much from this ability to press forward, to make new starts, to keep integrity intact in the face of loss and pain.

The women of Guatemala and El Salvador, like those elsewhere, tell me their birth stories. The vast majority of the women tell stories about the mid-wives who attended them at home, in their villages or towns. These midwives work for barter. I ask questions whenever time allows about the births of their first children, what the midwife did if there were complications, or who else assisted at the birth. My curiosity about the practices of midwives in Central America has been stimulated by the stories I hear in my clinic in Boston. I never would have predicted how moved I would feel as I sat and talked with older midwives—*parteras*—in Guatemala and El Salvador.

I traveled to San Salvador to participate in an international women's meeting with women representing many facets of Salvadoran life. In two days of meetings with the women's health care group, I had the honor of getting to know two older midwives from Chalatenango, one of the areas of El Sal-vador hardest hit by the war over the years. These women told stories of fleeing their burned villages to the refugee camps in Honduras, then return-ing to their villages to repopulate and reclaim the land from which they had been driven. In El Salvador, these women are regarded as criminals by the military because they are health promoters and are teaching people to take care of themselves. Each spoke with tears in her eyes about the lack of health care, the lack of clinics, how they had seen children die on the way to clinics where there would be no medicine waiting for them anyway. One told the story of running from the military during an attack while she assisted a woman having a baby. They ran behind a bush; the baby came; and both ran again; the mother holding her baby, bleeding and cord hanging, to safety behind a truck. She has watched women die from lack of medicine for hemor-rhages or for inability to pay a doctor who demanded fees prior to transport

to a hospital. I listened to them and thought how my tax dollars go to pay for the Salvadoran military's ability to keep repressing them, about their strength, their endurance, their will to survive.

Listening to them brought to mind the faces of the women from Central America whom I have had the privilege to care for in Boston. I knew I would go back to them different, angrier at the reasons for their pain, enriched by meeting the women who had cared for them in their own countries, and wanting to learn more.

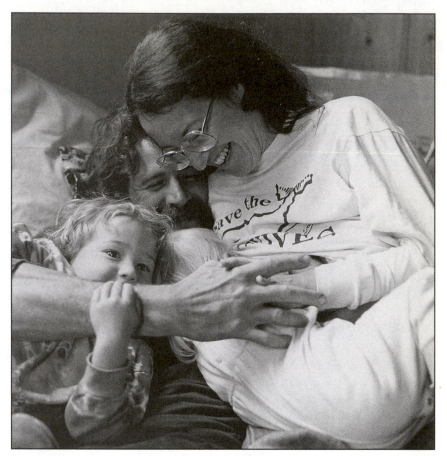

Jill Breen

A community midwife in rural Maine for seventeen years, Jill Breen has given birth to six children, all at home. Her midwifery training was in the apprenticeship mode and consisted also of self-study and participation in innumerable workshops on the differing philosophies of childbirth, midwifery, and health care. She has also been an emergency medical technician and uses herbs and homeopathy. She was on the board of directors of MANA for five years, speaks at colleges and workshops, and authors articles on midwifery philosophy and vision. A founding mother of Midwives of Maine (MOM), she lives on an organic fruit and vegetable farm with her family and attends births at homes in her community.

Jill Breen

I don't want to be their doctor, and I don't want to be a professional who's up above them, that's why I call myself a "community midwife." I want to be on an equal footing with my clients; I don't want their blood pressure to go up because they're coming to see me. I want us to be friends so they feel able to talk to me and know that I understand. We're looking at health and happiness as goals for their pregnancy and birth, and I want to help them achieve that. That's what I really like about being a lay midwife, that I'm the same as them.

When I had my first three kids, none of my friends had kids. Then when I had my fourth baby, I was finally having children at the same time as my friends. Now, in my forties, I have two new ones again, and the clients I am seeing are the same age as my daughter, and I have kids the same age as theirs. It's amazing that I'm getting to know a whole new generation of childbearing women. Our house is planned around the things we need and do. I even have the office near the front door and the bathroom, and I wouldn't know how to do midwifery any other way. It's a very personal thing for me, and so it's important that people know me and my family, my house, the chaos and everything. There's no way I would be able to work out of an office in town. I'm not interested in doing hospital births or birth center births. My philosophy of birth is my philosophy of life.

The [medical] backup situation for midwives [for problematic births] has changed a lot in the past ten years, and I'm pretty detached from it at this

point. With the backup relationships that I've had in the past, I've been unable to make my own decisions and was constantly having to battle the numbers: "What's her blood sugar? What's her blood pressure? What's her weight? What's her . . . ? What's her . . . ?" I like to risk people out on an individual basis, which includes considering how willing they are to work on things and how committed they are to having the birth go well. I've never transported anybody in terrible condition; I have a really good reputation. Part of my success is making sure that my clients know that they are the ones who are responsible for their well-being and their baby's well-being and I'm just there to help them. I've always felt that I'm there to help clients and not to assure the doctor that everything's cool and that all the medical issues are resolved. I'm there to help these couples do what they want to do as safely as possible. And I wouldn't have any compunctions about saying to someone, "I don't think this is a good homebirth situation," because the care you give is only as good as your honesty, and your love and the commitment of your clients. It has nothing to do with backup.

Birthing also has nothing to do with allopathic medicine. The best way to deal with something difficult is not necessarily to resort to drugs or knives. Sometimes midwives want to proceed in a certain way, but they can't because of hospital policy or the doctor backup situation. That's sad, and it's something I don't ever want to compromise myself about.

I also don't believe in third-party reimbursement for birth. Insurance policies are one of the major causes for the incredibly high rates of ultrasound and C-sections—it's because these interventions are covered by insurance policies. If they weren't, those frigging doctors would get their hands on the belly and figure out what's going on and deliver the kid for five hundred dollars and everyone could afford it. If midwives were covered by Blue Cross, Blue Shield and Medicaid, there's no way we'd be able to practice in the ways we want to practice, no way that we'd be able to do births the way people want us to do births.

We're much more open here in Maine about birthing policies; there's really no law. The attorney general's opinion is that pregnancy and birth are not medical conditions requiring medical care. That's why we can take care of women without being "medical practitioners." And this is a simple place for people to start—to get their medical practice act changed. The state has attempted to outlaw us a few times, but we've been able to catch up with them and testify at hearings. It becomes so obvious that doctors have their intense special interests and we don't. We're just doing our thing as safely as we can,

and this is what the consumers want. Consumers and midwives have civil rights, and we need to hold on to them because if we don't, they will be compromised right and left.

You keep having to put yourself out there, as a person and as a midwife, you keep having to say: "I believe in this," or "I really don't believe in that." Our standards have to be accountable to our values, not to the values of traditional medical practice in this country. For example, with the training of midwives, let's decide how a midwife should be trained, let's not try to be minidoctors. Let's decide how a midwife should be tested, and let's test her that way. Let's not kiss up to the standards of the medical profession in order to satisfy them that we are competent. Let's satisfy *ourselves* that we are competent. Intuition is often what makes us smart, what makes us do the work best, what makes us able to pick up problems earlier than anyone else and therefore deal with them more effectively. I don't think you can satisfy the medical establishment and be a midwife at the same time, I really don't.

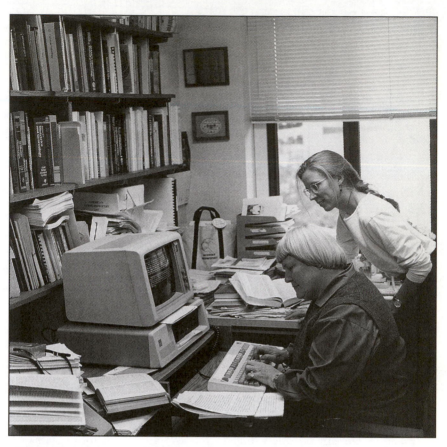

Helen Varney Burst

Helen Varney Burst, author of the first nurse-midwifery text in the United States, is a professor of nursing at Yale University. She has directed three nurse-midwifery programs. Her involvement in the ACNM has been extensive, including two terms as president, from 1977 to 1981. She has written extensively in the field of nurse-midwifery and has consulted for the development of many nurse-midwifery programs. She now serves as the chair of the ACNM Division of Accreditation and is currently conducting research for a book on the history of nurse-midwifery in the United States. She has recently inaugurated a column in the *Journal of Nurse-Midwifery* on historical perspectives, providing a place for CNMs to share memories, discuss what the past might mean to midwives, and record current events that will have significance in nurse-midwifery history. Besides her contributions to nurse-midwifery education, Burst is committed to enabling nurse-midwifery to make an impact on maternal and child health policy in the United States.

Helen Varney Burst

Everyone talks about being called to midwifery, but I had no such calling; rather, it was a progression from nursing, and even that was an accident too. Somewhere in my senior year of high school, I got out the college catalogue and ruled out just about everything except for nursing, because I didn't know enough about nursing to rule it out, so that's what I went into. I enjoyed nursing, and during my maternity nursing experience we used Ernestine Wiedenbach's book, which influenced a large number of nurses of that era to come into nurse-midwifery. She was a graduate in the 1940s in nurse-midwifery from the Maternity Center Association (in New York City) and probably coined the phrase "family-centered maternity nursing." I had a nursing instructor who had us experience a continuity of care type of situation, and I was on call to follow a woman through her labor and delivery. This was unusual in the framework of maternity care in 1959, when the medical center was still using twilight sleep [a state in which awareness and memory of pain are dulled or blocked; produced by an injection of morphine and scopolamine] with extensive use of forceps and spinals [a type of local anesthesia that causes numbing from the waist down].

But this did not happen with my patient—I sat with her. We breathed together, slept together through the night, and I was just smart enough to realize that when she started feeling the need to push that it was time to find someone else in the labor and delivery unit—it was night and everyone had kind of disappeared—to come for the birth. Well, that was my initial experi-

ence in maternity nursing, and it was the talk of the hospital, although I still didn't know anything about midwifery.

My instructor encouraged me to go on into maternity rather than psychiatric nursing or public health. She said, "You need to go and study under Ernestine Wiedenbach and you need to go quickly because she's about to retire." I had decided to teach on the undergraduate level, so when considering a graduate program in maternity nursing it was because I figured that I should know more than I expected my students to know. When Miss Wiedenbach asked me during my interview if I would be interested in nurse-midwifery, I asked what it was. She told me, and I said, "Sure, why not?" thinking that the more I knew, the better a teacher I would be. I thought that as a teacher you can effect more change than in individual practice. In individual practice you will affect the lives of the people you care for, but in teaching if I have ten students and in some way I affect their views and their philosophy in terms of standards of care and the facilitation of the natural process of birth then they will go out and affect all the women that they take care of, and you've multiplied yourself by tenfold. And if any one of those ten goes into teaching, then it becomes a ripple effect further and further out.

There's also the joy of watching the student grow and develop within the situation of learning about birth. To me, working with a woman and whoever she defines as family, and a student is an inclusive process, not an exclusionary process. And to me the midwife is there to facilitate others to be who they are. It has bothered me when midwives try to supplant the important others. We're but a moment in their lives—these other people will be their important people for a lifetime. So whatever we can do to make them be the important person in this significant process of childbirth is far more important than who I am in that particular situation.

When I was a student, we could do prenatal care, but it was legally questionable whether we could do labor and delivery in Connecticut, so we went to Kings County Hospital, a New York City hospital in Brooklyn, for the summer. At that time, the Maternity Center Association's nurse-midwifery program was there. There were two staff nurse-midwives, and the students and faculty from Columbia University and Yale University nurse-midwifery programs joined in the summer to obtain labor and delivery experience. My summer in Kings County was an eye-opener for me, facing a whole city of poverty and social problems. I went with a chip on my shoulder to try and change the system and was certainly naive and probably a nuisance.

When I graduated in 1963, there wasn't any place to practice nurse-

midwifery unless you came onto the staff of one of the few programs—there were only six of them at that time. So I went and taught undergraduate nursing in Wisconsin. After five years I went back to Kings County Hospital and was one of two Americans who ever took the family-training program run by United States Aid for International Development for foreign-trained midwives. I then did a nurse-midwifery internship to get back into practice. After my prior experience at Kings County Hospital, I decided that (1) I, particularly as a student, was not going to change the health care system in Kings County; (2) it would be a shame to do anything but learn everything I possibly could while there; and (3) I had learned somewhere along the line that, regardless of how bad the environment was, we can make a significant difference to that particular woman. So I focused on that and on learning and didn't fight the system, which was futile in the best of circumstances.

Family planning was illegal in Connecticut when I was a student. It was illegal to prescribe contraceptives or to use them, so our main function was to get women across the border to New York for family-planning methods. Family planning was legal in the New York City hospitals when I came back from Wisconsin. Before then we had to literally slip Planned Parenthood pamphlets underneath the sheet, and now we could counsel and prescribe oral contraceptives, fit diaphragms, and insert IUDs.

From there I went to Mississippi. I had been planning to go back to school and put together a mix of psychology and theology, but I didn't get accepted. The day I got my rejection letter a nurse-midwife who had been trying to recruit me to go with her to Mississippi on a federal project was elated and joyous because she didn't see any reason for me not to go now. There was—I didn't *want* to go to Mississippi. You finally ask that question, however, "What am I supposed to do?" and I felt very much that the Lord was telling me to go to Mississippi. So off I went.

The Mississippi project came about when Robert Kennedy took a swing through the Mississippi Delta area and saw things that appalled him—poverty, malnutrition, starving children—and he was deeply moved and went back to Washington, D.C., to do something about it. When Mississippi was invited to do something they set up a committee of nine within the state, which included the president of the white medical society, the president of the black medical society, the head of the health department, the head of the medical center, an all-purpose consumer representative, a minority woman, and three others. This committee actually did a very fine job, and somebody knew about nurse-midwives, so we got written into a three-part project. One

part was a nurse-midwifery education program in which the students would be funded by the federal government in return for a year of their life in the project. The second part was direct-care services, and the third was physician and hospital reimbursement so we could get our patients into the hospitals.

The first thing that happened to the project was that Robert Kennedy was assassinated and then the project suddenly got cut from two million dollars to one million dollars. The second thing was that we couldn't figure out why the federal funding agencies were so mad at us—we thought we were doing good things here and we were getting all this hostility. We found out later that the reason they were angry was the review process had been bypassed and that they were told they were going to fund us—period. Once we got into the system and started writing the grants things calmed down, and once we started being highly successful, things really turned around.

We had to decide early on what we were going to do in the whole area of civil rights. Were we going to be civil rights activists—which we all were but could we be in this situation? We made the decision to be very quiet, because the project could be killed instantly. We had to keep our eye on what it was we were trying to accomplish—and the bottom line was bringing health care to women and babies who because of poverty and racial discrimination were not getting it or what they were getting was totally inadequate. We made the decision to work within the system—within the health department. The reason was that if we could do it in one county then it could be replicated elsewhere. The health department in the South gave active health care in each county, unlike in the Northeast.

There was a nurse-midwife, Marie, who was originally from Minnesota and had spent her summers while in nursing school at a third-order Franciscan lay mission operation in Mississippi. She had become an activist when there was a very sick baby whose mother had tried to get into the hospital. The mother was black and could not get in, so Marie took the baby, she's white, and tried to get in and was refused access because the baby was black, and the baby died in her arms. She decided then to become a nurse-midwife and made a commitment to come back. She's the one who recruited me at Kings County.

So we were bound and determined to get the women into the hospital and decided not to do homebirths, which was where they gave birth because they had no other option. We were running into terrible sanitary conditions. We had people who were trucking in water from thirty miles away or had a well that was downhill from the outdoor privy. The windows had no screens,

and it was a real problem getting to many of our population who were living on backroads on plantations. There was a real problem of transportation in case of an emergency and then whether you could get them into the hospital. So our decision to do hospital births was based solely on getting them into the health care system, which would be positive for the population at that time.

There were originally six of us. Four of us were in Jackson to start the education program and run a nurse-midwifery service at the medical center. We had five counties we were supposed to cover with the other two midwives, so we started with one county as a demonstration project which could be replicated. But we didn't drop the other four counties—all six of us ran up and down the road to the clinics and did prenatal care and family planning but only did full midwifery practice in the one county.

The next thing we ran into was the racial tension. Two midwives who were friends came down from New York and assumed they would live together. One was black and the other was white. We were told in no uncertain terms that if they tried to live together they would be shot. It was as simple as that.

After we set up the demonstration project in Holmes County, the infant mortality was cut in half. We got the educational program off the ground, and our students dutifully served their time. We then expanded to a Southeast regional effort including the six southeastern states of Mississippi, Alabama, Georgia, South Carolina, Florida, and Louisiana. We sent our graduates out two-by-two to set up services across the Southeast. If you ever look at a map of how many nurse-midwifery practices there were before the Mississippi project and how many more there were after this got going—it was a significant increase.

The Mississippi educational program was closed in the mid eighties partially because it was federally funded and the funding ran out. The program was never well accepted in the very states' rights state of Mississippi (because they had civil rights forced down their throats), and they did not legislate the necessary funding to keep it going. Secondly, we came from the north of the Mason-Dixon line. I tried to say, "I'm from Kansas," rather than New York, but that didn't help, as it just conjured up images of John Brown at Harpers Ferry. Thirdly, I don't think one of us was a Baptist. Fourthly, we didn't think right in terms of much of anything. But the problem was not only the trust element from the white population but also the black population—they'd seen people come and go with their promises and then they were left as bad

off as they were before, if not worse because of dashed hopes. As I look back and say, "Well, were we like that or did we actually achieve something?" I'd like to think it's not just my biased opinion that we actually accomplished something that's everlasting in the provision of nurse-midwifery care through-out the South. So that was Mississippi—you can tell that was a powerful influence in my life.

In Mississippi we had developed a mastery learning curriculum utilizing modules [self-contained packets of materials that allow students to pace themselves individually], an approach that revolutionized nurse-midwifery education. Before we had the very traditional lecture approach—very straight-laced type of learning. A mastery learning curriculum basically says that in-deed any one person can learn, but you need to recognize that everybody has their own individual learning patterns. What you need is a smorgasbord of educational techniques and methodologies and to identify what the end-point objectives are and give students different ways to get there. As adult learners the students assume responsibility for their own learning, and you give them the tools with which to do this. How they achieve the learning objectives is their choice.

You can't insist that they come to class, for example, because maybe they don't learn that way. Maybe their time is better spent in the library. There is required clinical experience. Modules were set up by clinical compo-nents of antepartum, intrapartum, postpartum, and neonatal. This predated the core competencies outlined by the ACNM, and it revolutionized midwif-ery education to set down what we were actually teaching. I was on the initial examinations committee for the development of the national certification exam for the ACNM. The first thing we had to do was to define what we actually did—what in the heck is nurse-midwifery practice that we're going to test? Because it wasn't written down anywhere.

After teaching nurse-midwifery for five years and watching students struggling to put it all together, it was clear that there was a need for a book. I decided to write this book, and I figured that I couldn't direct a program and write a book at the same time. So I left and went to South Carolina to write it. I needed to get back to the ocean. I'm a water person, which is surprising, coming from Kansas. Before I finished I took over the directorship of the South Carolina nurse-midwifery program for a couple of years. I was now also president of the ACNM for two terms, and here I was preaching the good word of family-centered care, but where I was practicing didn't have it. The nurse-midwives had made tremendous inroads into the hospital but were

having terrible problems getting family into the labor and delivery area, and bed deliveries were still the exception, and they were facilitating breastfeeding over great obstacles.

The other thing that was happening in the 1970s was the whole development of lay midwives. And it was very clear to me in that setting from the chair of ob/gyn that homebirth would not be tolerated. And I knew that if any of us got involved in it, the nurse-midwifery program was instantly dead. And that was a problem for me because, as I said in my first presidential speech, I encouraged harmonious unity among nurse-midwives. There had been an uproar about homebirth versus hospital birth, and I was saying, "Hey, what are you talking about here? Our history is homebirth and we should be supportive and reinforcing of each other regardless of what setting we're in."

So here once again I was preaching something on the national scene and I could not practice that way in my own setting. It was a real problem for me. However, the purpose of this program was similar to Mississippi's, which was to produce graduates who would go out into South Carolina and bring health care to mothers and babies who weren't getting it, or what they were getting was less than adequate. We had to weigh whether to jeopardize our being able to bring health care to all these women against this issue of homebirth. So what I usually did was talk about these issues with the students who were eager to get into homebirth.

Then a lay midwife called a student from our program regarding a birth where the woman had torn and for whom she couldn't do the repair [suture the tear of the area around the vagina]. The woman was in the nurse-midwifery caseload for the student's prenatal care, and the student told the midwife to take her into the hospital and ask for the nurse-midwife. So here they came, mother, father, and baby, and unfortunately the nurse-midwife who was on call was young and inexperienced, not only in terms of her own capabilities technically but in terms of knowing how to manipulate a system. The first I knew of this situation was when I got a phone call about five in the morning saying that we might have a speck of trouble here.

And sure enough, the eventual pronouncement from the ob/gyn department was that we could no longer provide prenatal care to any woman that we knew was going to have a homebirth. And if a woman came to us and we found out in the course of delivering prenatal care that she was going to have a homebirth, we were to deny her care. This was on top of all the problems I was having with the dichotomy between what I was preaching and

with what I had to deal with—I couldn't do that. To me to deny care violated everything that I believed in so intensely, that there was no way I could do that. It was also the epitome of hypocrisy and racial discrimination. This mandate applied only to our very small private practice of white patients, while it was okay to continue to practice prenatal care and sign cards for the granny midwives to do homebirths for our black patients in the public health department clinics. I wouldn't live with this or be a party to it.

So that was the end of South Carolina for me. Eventually I had to leave—I had no choices because certainly I couldn't find a consulting physician who would back me up in any practice I would want to set up, in or out of the hospital. I was now a pariah and there was no one who would be associated with me at that time.

So I came to New Haven—coming back to Yale was coming home, as I graduated from here. I came back as the chair of the nurse-midwifery program—moving into my mentor's position. The school of nursing here has always been on the cutting edge of nursing, with very much a real sense of what a nurse can do in changing the health care system. In fact, this is the mission of the school—both by our practice and with being involved in policymaking and politics as well as the research. I initiated a course on public policy and women and infants. I didn't like the fact that nurse-midwifery students were graduating not knowing anything about the health care system, the way that maternal and child health is delivered within this country and the ways to use that particular system and work your way through it in order to get what you want for the women you are taking care of. I think that the public health emphasis is important. There's been a very close tie between public health and nurse-midwifery from the beginning of our history, so I would like to see that tie maintained, and reinforced. In New Haven the statistics for birth are as bad as Mississippi's were twenty years ago in certain census tracts within this city. We've got such terrible disparity between the black and white statistics—part of it is the problem of access to care and the kind of care you get once you access it, and we're trying to do something about it.

In the second edition of *Nurse-Midwifery* I put in a chapter on out-of-hospital birth, which included birth centers and homebirth. And I wrote another chapter on the collaborative management of complications, screening for high-risk situations which we then consult [with backup physicians on] and refer [to physicians]. In order to do this, because I won't write what I haven't done, I had to go learn about homebirths. I was co-founder of the

Family Childbirth Center here in New Haven. I also went to an inner-city hospital which was essentially a tertiary medical center run by midwives, in collaboration with doctors, where each woman who comes in is triaged, and the nurse-midwife will decide who else needs to get involved in the care of this woman. But regardless of risk status, regardless of complications, the nurse-midwife will continue with her no matter whoever else takes care of her, whatever the complications, so the nurse-midwife can still bring what normalcy she can to that birth.

In 1978 we had changed our definition in the ACNM of nurse-midwifery and of nurse-midwifery practice. The definition of nurse-midwife was clarified: that we belong to two professions, and that the nurse-midwife is educated in two disciplines—nursing and midwifery. One part of the definition of nurse-midwifery practice that changed was the inclusion of the words "independent management of care."

I gave a speech at the NAACOG [Nurses Association of the American College of Obstetrics and Gynecology] shortly after describing our new definition of a nurse-midwife, and it was the only place where I've ever spoken that I've gotten more applause at the introduction than at the end of my speech. I'd like to think it was because they were being very thoughtful, but I think it was because they didn't like what I had to say—basically that midwifery isn't nursing.

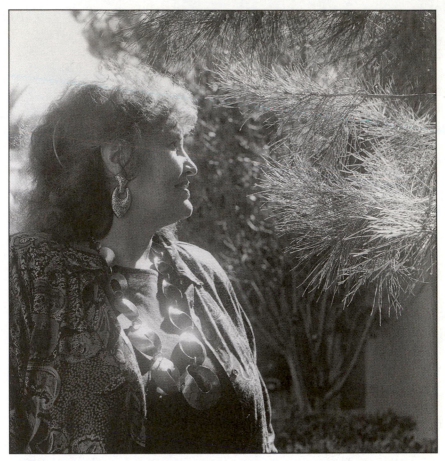

Barbara Cook

Barbara Cook has been working as a midwife for the past nineteen years and has attended over three thousand births. She has had a licensed birth center in Dallas for over fifteen years. For the past eight years she has taught an eighteen-week class on midwifery for the Texas Department of Health, and she administers and grades the midwifery exam for the Texas Department of Health. She received her initial midwifery training from the Maternity Center in El Paso, Texas, in 1976 and worked with a physician for four years, doing prenatals and births in the physician's clinic. She also teaches classes at North Texas School of Midwifery. Barbara is married to a man she describes as "very understanding" and has two children and three grandchildren, two of whom she delivered.

Barbara Cook

I had a friend who was having a baby and she was going to do it by herself. She wanted me to come and take pictures of the birth and just be there. But I got so excited when I was there that I didn't take pictures. After I had done hers, I went around in a daze, like I knew *that* was what I was supposed to do. Other people would come up and say, "Will you do ours? Why don't you do mine?" I didn't have any training, so I tried to find books to read. This was about 1975. So I started searching for books. The only thing that was out was Myles's textbook [Margaret Myles, *Textbook for Midwives,* 1981]. It was well over my head at that point. So I had a doctor who was doing homebirths show me how to do prenatal care, and then I would go out and labor sit for people. When they got to about six centimeters I would call him out, and he would come from his office to do the deliveries and I would be there watching. But then he got a lot of peer pressure for training midwives, so I went with another doctor who was seventy-three who delivered babies in the clinic. I'd go in and work for her some and cover for her when she went to Oklahoma. She taught me a lot and was more like a midwife than a doctor. Her name was Dr. Mayfield. When she retired, she gave me a bunch of her equipment—like her tables and her baby scale, which had probably weighed thousands and thousands of babies.

After I had been midwifing for six months, I found out that my great-grandmother was a midwife. She was a midwife out in Langtree, Texas. She

would go and stay a week or so with all the ranchers' wives and deliver their babies.

My own first birth was awful. It was back when they knocked you out. I labored all night long. I thought I was dying. Then they put me out and I didn't see my daughter for about eight hours. I was so groggy. They showed me the baby, and I didn't know if it was really mine or not. I had worked so hard for that. It was such a bad experience—I never got a chance to bond with her. It seems like her whole life we have tried to prove to each other that we really love each other. Then I decided that wasn't what I was going to do with my second one. When I got pregnant we were living out in western Texas. I stayed at home until the very last minute. I had my husband take me in. The baby was crowning and the doctor came in and gave me an epidural and held my legs together. But anyway I was awake and aware and I got to hold him. It was really something for the bonding process. Usually it is the daughter who is real close, but my son and I have always just had this bonding. It's not that I love my son any more, it's just that we don't have to prove to each other that we love each other.

My birth center is like a women's center, because they have a place to come and we make them feel welcome. They come in and get their herbal tea and sit around and have other women to network with and talk and they bring clothes. Other people come and dig through the box and get clothes. We have an "early-bird classroom," where they come in and get to meet other women who are early in their pregnancy. Afterward, because they get so close with us, they want to keep coming back even after they've had their babies. I've known women who got pregnant again just so they could come back into that atmosphere again. Then we have what we call a "materna-tea," where the women who have had their babies come back on the first Tuesday of every month. They sit around and make cookies, drink tea, and visit with people. It's really a nice atmosphere. You just feel good. It's not anything to have people call us when their kid's two years old and ask about the measles or this or that. They are good friends. You can't go anywhere in Dallas without somebody knowing you or recognizing you. It's a neat thing.

The kids come to the birth center along with their mothers for prenatal classes. They love to run to the water fountain, then to the toys. At the birth center I've got two exam rooms and two large birth rooms. One of the exam rooms could cover as an extra room if we had three in labor at the same time, which we rarely do. It's got a little day bed that you could deliver in if you

had to. Then there's a large living room and dining room. We've got three bedrooms, then we've got three apprentice rooms. It's an old Victorian-type house, just real homey looking, real frilly. It's got the windows and French doors and stuff. It's a nice old house, but it's like every old house you know, there's always something to do on it.

I see my role as letting the women do birth their way. I've been with other midwives that try to push or are playing doctor. I like to lay back and let them do it their way. Some women want to lay in bed. I've seen some people say, "Get out of bed! Walk and it will go faster." I tell them to listen to their own bodies. What their bodies are usually telling them to do is what is best for them. You may make suggestions, reminders like, "You may need to empty your bladder," or this or that. But as far as trying to fit anybody into a certain way, I don't. I think everybody's an individual. It's *your* birth. We have some people who bring a whole bunch of people. They are happy with that. Some people just want me and their husband there. Or they just want nobody but them and their husband until the very last minute. Then we come in. As long as it's safe, anything they want to do with their birth is their business. Who they want to have there, whoever makes them feel comfortable.

I really see birth as a normal happening now. I've seen a lot of complications. I think the body compensates for itself in a lot of areas. I don't think that it is dangerous, or I wouldn't be doing it. If it were really dangerous, I just wouldn't do it. If there's a problem, I'm the first one to say, "Look . . . ," and we're out the door. The baby is here long after the birth. Where they have the baby is really not that important, as long as it's a safe and healthy baby. I'm not going to sit around and fool with heart tones dropping to eighty or below. Even though we're that close to the hospital, I don't take the chances. I'm just there for the birth. These people are going to have to deal with their babies the rest of their lives. I'm not going to allow one to become brain damaged because I have this ego problem about going to a hospital or something. I always tell people to plan to have it the way they want to. We have a birth plan that they make out that says who they want, if they want special music, or they want a special gown or some sort of a ceremony. It's their birth plan and at the bottom of it, it says, "What if the unexpected happens?"

We just tell them to have a plan A and a plan B and not to feel like they're a failure or anything—if plan A doesn't go through, we just move to plan B, which would be to transfer to the hospital. We say this is happening right now, and this could become a problem and this could happen. For

example, if she starts running a little temperature or something, we say, "This could be the first sign of an infection. If that happens, we'll have to go in. We'll keep a watch on it," and that type of thing. We keep them informed so she knows what's happening. The father, too, so that they can make decisions together. If there is a transport we usually give them a few minutes to get used to the idea. We say, "This is happening and we may need to move into a hospital. That might be in ten or fifteen minutes." And give them time to settle it out.

I never attend a birth by myself unless it's an emergency. I would guess through my career I've probably attended thirty or forty births by myself. I have one or two apprentices with me all the time. I really don't like to take apprentices who have small children, because I feel like part of our goal is to be building happy families. So to have an apprentice with real small children, it kind of rips the family up because they're gone so much. I see that many midwives are so young. I guess they balance things out by not doing so many births. If they do one birth a month or something, then they can handle it. But apprenticeships like those at our birth center are really intensive. We do prenatal care three days a week, childbirth classes on Friday nights, then you have to be there for births. We do fifteen or sixteen births a month—that's like one every other day. It's all-consuming. They have to be at all the births and all the prenatals, so that people get to know them. You don't want strangers at people's births. It's really a hectic pace.

My husband is a computer programmer. He does his thing and I do mine. Then we get together and enjoy each other. My kids are pretty well grown. My son was about sixteen or seventeen when I started. My husband fends for himself. He does things around the birth center if I can't get a handyman. When my husband hears of other women getting sued or different things, he worries. But I think he's pretty proud. The other day I heard him talking to someone and he said, "Yeah, I'm known as Mr. Barbara Cook." I guess it was his way of giving a compliment. When we start arguing, we know we haven't been together enough. It's time for a trip. We have a lot of friends that have nothing to do with midwifery. That's kind of how you balance it. When you walk away from the center you just cut it off until the phone rings, then you go back there again. I have a beeper all the time. My home's about twelve minutes away from the birth center. When I'm there it's all-consuming, but when I walk out I shut the door. It took a while to learn how to do that. There are other things in life, like travel. I just love to travel. I love to be with my friends.

The uncertainty of the hours is probably the hardest part of midwifery. You never know when somebody is going to call you. Sometimes you're so tired after being out for two or three days and finally you get to go home. I always go in and take a nice warm shower from head to toe—I just kind of wash off the births behind me. I crawl in bed and when the phone rings again I just feel like crying, "No, I can't do it!" You always have to act happy for them. "Oh, you think you're in labor. Great! Well, I'll meet you over there." You drag out of bed and go back over there for another twenty-four hours. You always keep telling yourself even on a real long labor, it will always be over at this time tomorrow and I'll get to rest. That's how you get through— one day at a time.

Transports are really hard. I hate to take someone in because I want them to have the kind of birth they want, and it's real hard for them to get that in the hospital. But doctors are much better now than they used to be. When I first used to take people in on a transport, they would act like I was trying to kill them. Doctors would rant and rave at me for hours.

They know now what a midwife is. When I first started nineteen years ago it was real hard. It was not only the doctors, but the mothers and the mothers-in-law. They would all act like you were trying to kill their grand-children. Their kids were crazy hippies and that kind of stuff. So we had to do a lot of convincing. Now you don't have to, because my reputation kind of stands on its own. I've done over three thousand births. They know it can be done. Everybody knows somebody that's had a homebirth. Back then they had never heard of it. It's a lot easier now than it used to be. When I first started they weren't even allowing fathers in the delivery room. In fact, down in Georgia a man handcuffed himself to his wife because he wanted to be with her. It was in the newspaper. They called the sheriff's office to kick him out of the delivery room. Just think, what would it hurt for him to be with his wife? Then they called the sheriff to go put him in jail for wanting to be with his wife. It's ludicrous. What made them gods? What made them the guardians of our bodies and our babies?

I'm not against all doctors. I'm the first one to take somebody in if it's beyond what I can do. I just hate the whole system. It's just not right. The doctors down in Central America, Mexico, and Guatemala, they don't think they're gods. They are there to serve the people, and in most instances they don't make too much more money than the average person. Here it's like they're gods or something.

I love it when the baby comes out and you give it to the mother. I love

their joy. You could ask some eighty-year-old woman, "What happened on your first birth, or your second or your third?" and she could remember every detail. "Well, Paw was out in the field plowing and my water broke," and this and that. It's a highlight in a person's life. To get to be there and share it and make it a special moment for them is really great. To feel good about it and feel good about themselves. It's just a wonderful, wonderful moment. I just love doing it.

I believe that nobody could be an atheist after seeing a birth, because you know that God's hand is in the birth process. The body is such a beautiful, wonderful working machine. I don't know how anybody could think of evolution or anything else when you see what's happening. I know there's a lot of different types of midwives and some of them are very religious and want to pray over all their clients. I think—and I really do have strong religious beliefs—that people don't come to me for my religious beliefs or for me to preach to them. There are midwives that do that. I think they come to me for my skills. I have very, very poor people, they're almost street people, that come in. They love me as well as my rich people. There are some times you can just come in and laugh and just have a ball with your clients. Then there are some that expect you to be so dignified. You just have to be intuitive to what each one wants out of you as a midwife and just fulfill it. I've been able to do it, because I have such a varied clientele. It's neat. I enjoy getting to know the people. We've got Hare Krishnas and Christian Scientists who won't take a vitamin pill. You just have to go along with their belief system. You just have to respect each person as an individual, their lives, their religions as well as food. We have a lot of people eating junk food and then we have vegetarians. I think you have to let the whole person go along with their belief system. Some people really want a mother, a person to hug them, and be sweet with them. Some people want you to be strong. Sometimes people even like you to lecture at them: "Look at you, you've only gained three pounds. You better gain some more weight." That kind of stuff. You just have to know the individual and what they like from you, and do it. It's pretty easy after doing it for so many years. Sometimes you can kid them out of it, or sometimes I'll hold them and they'll cry a real lot and open up. Everybody that comes to me gets used to getting hugs. They won't leave without a hug. One of the girls at the desk will say, "Didn't I get your appointment?" and they'll say, "Yes, but Barbara hasn't come to give me my hug yet."

Then there's some people that are real standoffish at first. I'll go over to these rich, rich houses to do homebirths. They're real dignified people.

You just act dignified and see what they need and move into that role. You just have to be able to know what they need and give it to them.

We do a lot of underwater births. We've got a portable hot tub, and then we've got the big old type of bathtub, with the claw feet. A lot of people deliver in that. I did my first water birth three-and-a-half years ago. They did an article in a Dallas magazine on us doing underwater births. There are more and more clients asking for that. Almost all of our people labor in water and then a lot of times it just kind of happens. They don't plan a water birth, but then they just don't want to get out. We'll just say, "Do you want to stay here?" "Yeah? Can I?" and we just bring the equipment into the bathroom. Or if they really want a water birth, we fill up the portable bathtub, which is really big, with water and sea salt.

One lady was in labor for thirty-six hours. She was a psychotherapist and a single mom. She looked like a drowned rat. She didn't get out of that tub for thirty-six hours practically, just to get up and go to the bathroom, or to put more hot water in. She kept the birth room real dark and she kept the music going. It was like she was just floating through time and space. She was real small and had a nine-pound baby for her first baby. She was one that they wrote up in the magazine. She probably would have had a C-section in the hospital. As long as it's safe they can do anything they want to. But there's so many people that have different ideas. You just have to be understanding and respectful of other people's ideas. It's their business and their right as a person to believe the way they want to and birth the way they want to.

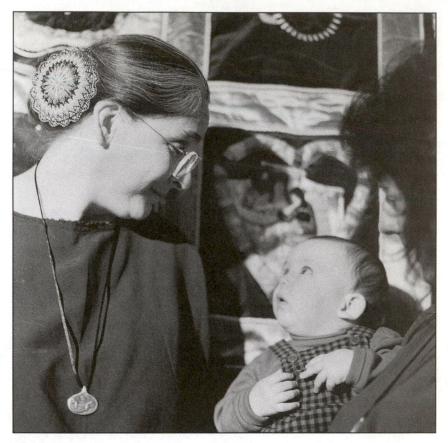

Mary Cooper

Mary Cooper is an apprentice-trained midwife who has been serving the Amish community in Ohio for the past ten years. Mary was the midwest regional representative to MANA and has been a popular speaker both at MANA and Midwifery Today conferences. Her experience in hospice work with the dying gave her the background to lead workshops on grief, and she also speaks frequently on vaginal birth after cesarean (VBAC) and twin births. Mary is also an EMT. She believes that birth is sacred ground onto which midwives need to tread with utmost respect. Her Christian devotion is central to her practice of midwifery. Mary has two daughters, one whom she attended in labor, another one who is interested in becoming a midwife and has begun to learn the skills; and a son with Down's syndrome, who has been one of her special teachers. She recently has taken a sabbatical to recuperate from her many years of service.

Mary Cooper

I got into midwifery because I was a twenty-year-old single woman who was pregnant. The father of the baby was in Vietnam. He wasn't going to be out by the time the baby was born. I found out [about the pregnancy] when he had just gotten six weeks into being in Vietnam. I worked in a hospital in orthopedics. I thought, Well, it's okay, I'm young, I'm strong. I had already started collecting midwifery books, birth books, and things like that. I wanted to have my baby at home, and I didn't think it would be a problem, because I was an employee at the hospital. I thought my wishes would be more respected than the common person coming in off the street because they would know me, and they would bend over backward to help me do that. I said no medication, no pitocin [a synthetic hormone that induces or enhances labor contractions], don't cut my bottom, no drugs, no forceps, and I want to have my mother there. My doctor said no problem.

When I went into labor at about three centimeters, they hooked me up and the contractions got hard real soon. They sent my mother down and I never saw her again. I could hear her out there fighting to get in. There was nobody else in labor. The nurses' station was right outside my room. I didn't see another soul for five hours. During a contraction at one point, a nurse came in and stuck a hypodermic full of Demerol into my thigh. I was squatting in the bed, and they would come in and tell me to stop. That's where they discovered me five hours later. What I didn't know is that I had a pitocin drip, and five hours later I thought, well maybe this is bigger than I am.

Maybe this is harder. Maybe I really can't do this—I could just have a cocky personality. What I didn't know was that I was eight centimeters and going into transition, because I didn't have anybody there.

So they took me to the delivery room. They found me squatting in the bed and just about had a hissey. So they took me into the delivery room. They told me to curl up on my side, and they did a caudal [local anesthesia]. I was numb from the waist down. I didn't realize what they were doing. I just did what they told me to. So I couldn't push, and when I couldn't push, I ended up having a very long, deep episiotomy into my rectum, and had high forceps. I didn't realize. My bottom didn't hurt then. I was just so happy to see my eight-and-a-half-pound daughter that it didn't matter. Then later on, I started thinking about it. I thought, this guy really lied to me. I knew exactly what I wanted. There was no reason for me not to have my baby at home. They were more worried about the fuss my mom was making, or that I wasn't for publication in the newspaper, because I was an unwed mother. I thought I would never do that again.

I knew that birth should be natural. I had an intuitive instinctual feeling that birth would be okay. I'm a big person; I'm 5'10''. I've worked hard. My body is good. My mother had twelve children. She never had any trouble having babies, even though she had a face presentation, two breech babies, and two sets of twins. She said, "You can do it." I'm a pretty big, strong woman. My next labor, twelve years later—Ananda was a fifty-minute labor from start to finish. I get to about six centimeters and pop, the next contraction she's pushing out. Then Ian was a thirty-seven-minute labor start to finish. My husband was there for Ananda's birth. He and I did it ourselves. I just talked to him instead of breathing, 'cause the contractions started transitional type when the labor started. She had come so quick, she had sucked a gulp of water down. I had a DeLee [suction device to clear the baby's throat and windpipe] beside me and I suctioned her. With Ian, Ananda sat right beside me. She was almost three years old, and patted his head as he crowned and said, "This is my baby coming."

After my first baby, I was trying to join the Peace Corps but I was rejected because I was a single person with a child. About this time I heard about midwives, and I tried to find them. I had gathered a whole lot of books and started really reading. I was a grassroots person. I worked in the free clinic. I have almost always been in a co-op for good food. I got into a structured program administered from Columbus, Ohio, apprenticed there for twenty months, worked with a homebirth doctor for a year, but basically

went out on my own. I live in a homeschooling area, natural, homeopathic, herb, rural. I am a community midwife. I live in the community and I help the families in my community. My community extends forty-five miles. It's close. I'm on the edge of an Amish community and I work with four Amish communities and two Mennonite communities. Every Monday and Thursday I go to six different places to do prenatal care. There's always four Mondays in a month. The Amish will usually write me a letter [since they don't have phones] and they know which day of the week I come to their community and they say, "Put me back on the list. My last period is this. I think I'm due here." I go to their farms. I've done twelve prenatals in a day. One day we did fifteen.

My English couples, they come to my house, where I see them in our living room. My family works around the schedule. We do baby and prenatal care three to four days a week, then home visits and follow-up visits, especially if there's a special-needs child that we need to follow up on, or somebody calls me out because somebody cut themselves and I need to do stitches on them, or check out this rash. I check out blood pressures on the elderly people in the community. I do hospice care and have worked with our local EMT service. I don't ride squad anymore, but I use the training just in everyday life. If there is an emergency, this training helps me recognize it. I believe in serving the public if you can. I really believe in that. I believe in helping people, sharing knowledge, being—for lack of a better expression—an elder, and giving back. You can give back through knowledge, and helping the young folk.

We do, on an average, ten births a month. The least we've ever done is six and the most we've ever done is twenty-one in a month. I'm a very strong-minded person. I can tell that I'm very deeply tired right now. I rely on the strength of the people I help. I rely on the strength of the Lord, who says, "Nothing is impossible," and that he won't give you more than you can do. I know that I probably read into that as far as, I don't say no to people. I just can't pick and choose and say, "Well, I can help you, but I can't help you." I just can't do that. There are things that I let go. I used to be a room mother at school. I used to do squad work. I used to be a hospice worker. Now, if they really need me, I will do it, but it's not something that I do weekly or monthly like I used to. We still do a very big organic garden. Ananda and I still put things up. We do a lot of freezing. A lot of the births that I do are at night, so I come home and I just give up a day of sleeping. I do what I have to do and just go to bed earlier. I'm a real strong-minded person. This is exactly

what I want to do. I am tired. It would be nice if I had somebody to work with, but I don't, so . . .

My daughter Ananda wants to be a midwife. She has gone to births with me, goes to prenatal care with me. She writes down the blood pressure and the pulses and she's the one already calling it to my attention. "Well, Mom, the last blood pressure was this," or, "Her pulse is up a little bit," and whatever. She's ready, she's lived it since she was born. She was ten days old when I went back to the practice and now she helps me. When there's people that have come to the house to have their babies, Ananda has cooked, or she does whatever, or she watches Ian while I'm with the woman. It's ingrained in her. I tell her she needs to give back. When you get knowledge, you share it, you give it back, or it's wasted. You pass it on. For lack of a better expression, you're a servant.

I have a midwife's back from bending over, trying to get a baby to nurse, being with a woman or squatting or laying down or being in a position to twist to accommodate her birthing position. I have a very sore lower back. I can tell it. I can't hang people [have them put their arms around her neck and hang from her during a labor contraction] like I used to for hours—hold them up as they hang their weight. It's taken its toll some. I go to a chiropractor periodically, and Ananda gives me a back massage. I'm a real bulldog.

Ian is my seven-year-old son, and he's Down's [syndrome]. I am so thankful that I have Ian; he is my teacher. He had a whole lot of allergies. We put a lot of time into this little boy, because he was really sick the first two years of his life. For a while, he had such severe allergies that there were about only eleven things that he could eat, and three of those were herbs. We belong to the largest cooperative in Ohio, and the co-op truck comes and we unload it for four hours. We get organic, nonpreservative fresh fruit that we use. We pretty much just cook from scratch. It's really pulled Ian around. He's a different little boy. Nutrition is pretty important to us. He still has a lot of allergies. He has what we call a Down's bowel. He just does not absorb certain foods, but he's real healthy. It's a priority.

Ananda has been homeschooled for two years. She went to the regular school, per her choice, for three years, kindergarten, first, and second grade. Then she asked us to be at home. We call it car school, since we do so much of it on the road. Ananda is pretty disciplined. A lot of the schooling is by herself. When she was nine, she was doing meals. She knows how to sew. She's the seamstress of the family. There was the one year that she did three or four of her own dresses. They were simple, but she did them. She reads a

lot. She is very creative and she's a real gentle soul. She's been good and Ian has been the teacher for that. He teaches patience. Ian is a teacher. All of our children are teachers, but having a special child has taught us patience, a certain amount of courage and seeing through.

Sometimes I've got this situation that has suddenly popped up and I just think, Can I handle this? and this life is in my hands. It's just an awesome responsibility. It is something that is always there. An aspect of my practice that is incredibly important to me is that I feel it is a ministry. It's a ministry to anybody who would walk through my door. I don't particularly turn anybody away. I've only, I think, said no to five or six people in fourteen years. That was because a couple of people smoked and they wouldn't stop, or a couple said, "I'm coming to you because you're cheap." I said, "No, that's not why we have babies at home." I am definitely nurtured and appreciated by the community in the work that I do. I love what I do, love it.

I have also done hospice work—life is very precious. There's a lot to learn from it. We just have to open ourselves up to it. Sometimes there are aspects to our lives that bring us pain. I've always thought that it is through pain that we get our biggest insights into life, and learn the most. You just have to humble yourself to the lesson that is there. It can't be our way sometimes. You can't hurry it along, or say, "I need" or "I want this." Sometimes the message is right there in front of our face and we don't see it. We've told my mom, "You can come live with us anytime you want, because the other aspect of birth is death." My mother wants to always be at home to die among her family, and for it to be a family member's voice the last thing that she hears before that life's spark is gone. I believe in that. I believe in that community, that family. And I rest assured that my daughter will help me and help take care of me in my old age. That's important.

I've had babies that it took me a little while to get them started. I pray. I ask the Lord to guide my hands, to just bless my hands and tell me what I should do, when I'm thinking that there is something wrong. There's been plenty of times, just numerous times: I can remember the first time I ever had to cut a baby's cord that was around the baby's neck. I don't know why I opened those packages and my sterile instruments to have them ready, because I wouldn't have had time. I heard this voice that said, "Watch the cord. Watch the cord. It's around the neck." So I just got everything ready, and it was a very short cord and it was around the baby's neck. It was so tight the baby's face was white. As soon as I clamped it and cut it, the baby came and it was fine. We all have those times when heart tones [the baby's heartbeat as

monitored by fetoscope] aren't rebounding as well as you want, and you just say, "Something's up. Something's up. Something's up." You have this little nagging voice that says, "Pay attention. Pay attention." You don't know why you're paying attention, but you're more aware. Your ears are fine-tuned, your hands are real, you're going to take heart tones a little more often; it's that voice of instinct.

My daughter Jennifer when she was eighteen had a frank breech baby at home. It was good, because I knew what Jennifer's alternative was. They would have cut her, she would have had a cesarean. My daughter has an absolute zero pain tolerance. Unfortunately, her water broke early, so it didn't cushion her as much as it should have. It was tough on her. She didn't like it when it came time—she dilated very quickly like I did. Her water broke at midnight and she had the baby at 7:20 in the morning. When it came time to push, she just gave these little grunt pushes like, "Uh, uh. Okay, I'm pushing. Uh." It came time and she said, "Mom, I want this baby out." I said, "You have to do more than that. You can do it." I don't do very many internals—I suspected that he was breech all along, but I never did an internal. Therefore, it wasn't confirmed. The baby was so low in the pelvis anyway. There came a time when she was in transition. The baby was pushing her bones, and it hurt her. She looked up at me and said, "Help me Mom. Help me." You know it was like, "Save me." That disarmed me for a little while. I wanted to just go and cry, to give her the strength, or just do it for her. I went in and washed my face and said, "Oh God, just be with me, and give her the strength to do it." I went in and woke my husband up and said, "This is really hard on her." He said, "You can do it. She's in good hands." About five minutes later he got up and said, "I'm going into work early." I thought, You chicken. She did it. She delivered a six-pound, ten-ounce frank breech baby over an intact perineum.

She hadn't wanted to have babies right away. She didn't even want to deliver at home. She told me, "I'm going to have my baby in the hospital, 'cause they can give me drugs." I later said, "Why did you want to have your baby here?" She said, "Mom, those were all words, until I had to make a decision, until I found myself pregnant." She said, "I realized I had to be with somebody who loved me and really cared for me, and wouldn't hurt me, someone I could trust." She says that if she ever had another baby, she would stay at home.

I never confirmed to her that the baby had stayed breech. She wanted the baby to have hair, because all the Cooper babies had always had hair. She

would say, "Does it have hair, Mom?" and I would say, "No." She would say, "Do you see the baby's head?" and I would say, "I see the baby." She would have frozen if she had known the baby was breech. When the baby was born, she reached down and took the baby. She looked at me and said, "You lied to me," and I said, "Ya, you're right, the baby was breech." She said, "No, no, no, he's got plenty of hair." It's the only time in my career almost, that I ever didn't tell someone the truth. I lied. She said, "I'm glad you didn't tell me it was breech, because I would have frozen. I would have never been able to do anything." I just knew that. That's how the kid is.

I was firm in the church until I was about seventeen. I left it for a while. I came back to it, because I firmly believe that you have to have a faith. How can you be a midwife and not believe in God? Birth is bigger than we are. It's just bigger. Birth is a miracle. It's just a miracle. Over and over again, every time I see a baby born, I'm just awestruck. Especially with the courage you see from women. Women are so courageous. I see some real brave women. They know that it is going to hurt. They think that they can't bear it, but they want those babies and they're going to do it. They submit to whatever the birth journey is going to be. I'm just truly amazed. I'm amazed by bodies that give to let babies out. I'm amazed by the courage that some women have to get those babies out. For some women it is hard to have a baby. I don't know where people think that strength and miracles come from. Where does that little voice come from that tells us what to do sometimes, or to be aware of? Or, you're afraid because a certain situation comes up and there is a decision to be made. You can almost feel the pulse that is there. That is, "It's okay. It's okay." Or, to give a woman courage when a doctor is trying to induce them, because she is so late, and you just know. You just know in your bones that baby hasn't cooked enough [isn't due to be born yet]. It just hasn't put enough weight on, and that everything is okay. You turn around and validate her knowledge and courage to just wait it out a little more. Or you have a mother whose belly's been cut twice from having cesareans, and she just wants a vaginal birth so bad. You know it's okay. It's the mother asking you to respect her courage and her claims. You just feel this voice, "This really is okay. This woman really can do it." I want to be there to help her. I want to be there to support her, because she has to have even more courage. She has a lot of people, people who honestly love her, who are afraid for her to try to attempt to have a vaginal birth after a cesarean. But she knows that she can do it, that she's strong and her body will hold up. She

wants it. In some ways we're going along as the helpers, to help that person achieve that.

I have had to work real hard for the doctor backup that I have. For the most part the doctors are very respectful. We refer people back and forth. Some of the doctors I get my medicines from. With one in particular, maybe the couple only sees him once and he says, "Fine, if you're working with Mary, that's great. If you run into problems, call me. I will meet you at the hospital." I go in with my people. I'm not just going to drop them off at the door. Even if I could possibly get some flak. That's not fair. I have gotten flak, as far as I had a city law director who said, "You're practicing illegally. You're practicing medicine without a license." I just try not to be stupid. Also, if something happened and I needed to go in, I would. It's being responsible, and it's seeing my commitment through. I'm a big believer in commitment.

I have had some students in my practice but they just didn't understand the sacred ground. I'm a real believer that birth is sacred ground. One woman in particular, I would say, "You can come in the room, when you can see the head, if you need something." She would just stand in the doorway with her mouth open and gape. I said to her, "To me you are like a voyeur. You are an intruder. This was a privilege that this woman invited you to this birth to learn. You are disrespectful." Not all the students are like that. I have had apprentices who have said, "You're just so busy. I just don't want to be this busy." I think my practice is overwhelming to a lot of people. I have a lot of people who say, "I can't keep up with you. I can't keep up with your kids." It's sort of a way of life.

I try to ask the babies to be respectful. It is my prayer that babies come one at a time, in their own time, and bless the hands that will be there. Don't bless my hands in particular, but bless the hands that will be there. If it's the mom's hands, the dad's hands, the sister's, the child's, another midwife's, just bless the hands that will be there. Just be there with those hands—and have the babies come in their own time.

I do a lot of births for nothing. If there is a transport, I don't charge anything. If the parents want to give something back, that's fine, but then I think of the hospital bill. I do a lot of births for free for poor people, some of the poor families that I know, or the struggling families. I barter a lot. I've bartered winter wood. One year when my corn crop failed, the husband of one of my clients called me up and said, "We have some corn for you." I had just seen him two days before, and I had asked him to save me two dozen ears

for eating, so I thought he was talking about that. I was pretty tired, and he goes, "No, you must come today." I said, "Okay." So, it was about thirteen miles away. I went, and Katie, his wife, and the two oldest girls had taken thirty dozen ears of corn and shucked it, desilked it, cut it off the cob, and I had twenty-five quarts of corn there to put up. That was great. I've gotten four or five calves for what I do. I got a registered Nubian goat once. It was gonna have kids. I've gotten quilts and I've gotten beautiful sets of bookcases made. Sometimes there's a loaf of bread stuck in between my doors, a dozen cookies. I've gotten a pie. I've gotten a bushel of green beans. I feel blessed. I like what I do. I hear at least once a month, "Mary, I don't know what we'd do without you." Or, somebody will introduce me and they will say, "This is *our* Mary." I'm real blessed, real blessed. I'm lucky I have them. They give me a purpose to my life. I get to do what I really like. If I don't get paid, that's cool. It's part of my tithing of giving back to the community. Even my largest fee isn't very much, and I just raised it. It's anywhere from zero to five hundred fifty dollars. That's it for everything.

The Amish aren't as afraid of birth as the English are. They really just open up and say, "Well, I'll take what I get," in terms of the kind of labor. "I hope I can do it. It's okay. I know it's hard work, but look what I get." They love their babies. They know. They're definitely much shier and more modest, but they know how it's going to be. It's part of their culture to have a lot of babies. I've seen a lot of bravery, courageousness. They have a faith that if a child is lost or something happens, that child is in a better place. That child is already healed in the Lord's hands. They have more of an understanding, if you make a mistake, if you make a judgment call, and call it wrong and something through a twist, or through a precipitous birth, or something that maybe happens that you make a mistake.

There was one birth where the mother suddenly went into polyhydramnios [excessive amount of amniotic fluid]. You couldn't palpate, and the baby's movement was going down. I just thought, This has got to be a special baby. Something is going on, and it was. It was a Down's baby with multiple abnormalities. I think that if it had twelve, twenty more hours, it would have been a uterine death, a stillborn baby. It was actually hard to have this little seven-pound girl. She just wasn't drinking the water anymore. That is why the water was building up. I worked on the baby, listened, did mouth-to-mouth [resuscitation], and the baby was already semirigid. I said, "Rosey, Melvin, I don't think this baby can make it." They said, "We don't want you to do that. We just want to hold her for the time she has." That would be a

decision I would make, personally. I wouldn't want somebody to save my baby that had no life. You could tell that this baby was going. It wasn't going to be with us much longer. They were actually surprised that she lived for twenty minutes.

They have much more of an acceptance. I'm accepted. They are very reality-based as far as that every child that is conceived is not meant to be with you. They know forgiveness. Last year, last August fifth, my Amish community was in the news when a drunk driver hit a buggy that had eleven people in it; seven were killed. It was from the same family. They had just come back from celebrating a birthday party, and eating cake and ice cream. A mom, several sisters and a son-in-law, and several of the children were killed. It was horrible. They called me up and said, "Come down. We want you to come down and be with us," and I did. They wanted me to come to the funeral, to the viewing, and to be there. They were very upset, and this man was charged with manslaughter, because they had forgiven him. They had. They said, "We forgive him a hundred times, a hundred." The county prosecutors prosecuted him for six vehicular homicide deaths. He received six years. They said, "We're not this man's judge and jury. He has to live with the fact that he has taken these lives and that we forgive him. There may be a time when someone will need to forgive us." There was one time when the health department got a little upset with me, and I had two of the Amish fathers call me and say, "If you need our support, we're there."

I think it is very important to let women know how strong they are, and how brave they are to have babies. Sometimes they will be faced with birthing situations they wouldn't ask for. The support is so important. Education, the traditional route to me is just so important that it be passed down. It is important that we, as the elders, help the young women coming up in the ranks, help the children to pass it on. I think it is imperative. I think it is important to work with all aspects of the family. For us to understand that we are only as good as the people that come through our doors and ask our help. Where would we be without the round tummies that walk through our door?

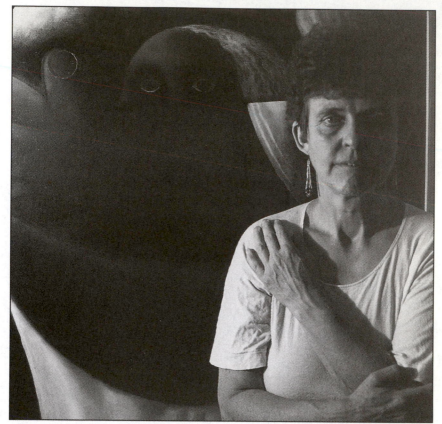

Trudy Cox

Trudy Cox was raised in the northeastern corner of Oregon in the mountains, in part by a horse and some dogs. She attended Georgetown University to become a nurse-midwife and later got a degree in community health/public health from the Northeastern University School of Nursing. She has worked in several hospitals in the Boston area and has attended homebirths as well with independent midwives. Trudy worked in a rural birth center in Zimbabwe in 1988, attending births and educating midwives there. She is a mother to "two wonderful adult children who are all she could hope for." She is not sure what she wants to be when she "grows up," but it must involve the outdoors, rocks, water, acting, and singing. Justice is important to her.

Trudy Cox

In labor I was alone. When I was wheeled into the delivery room there was a black Jamaican midwife, who left me alone and kept her distance from me. I've had all these years to think back through my birth experience in Jamaica again and again. There were years when I felt abused by that, but now I think it was a rare and good experience to be left by myself to birth that baby. No help of any kind. It's a strange experience, but it is an aspect of midwifery that I appreciate, to just leave birth alone. Because I do not control people, I refuse to control people. Somehow that got in here when he was born.

I howled—I can hear myself howling when he was born and I knew that my just giving birth, alone, on my own, really was the best model of midwifery that I have ever seen or participated in. All through these years I've said that I am going to figure this out and then I'll be done with it. That's what I'm looking for—to only be present and facilitate while women do this thing. My role should be so minimal that I'm only there as a safety factor.

I get the feedback, especially from men, that what's really strange about my practice is that I am willing to let something happen the way that it happens. The world of obstetrics thinks that that's incredibly dangerous. Somebody might die if you just let things happen. They don't ever use that sense of just being present. They don't think like that—ever, to not do anything that's not necessary. Because there is only one person who has any kind of control in the situation—which is the woman. But the doctors don't really get it that that's true.

114

At home you have the strength of the environment to help with birth. You have the intimacy, the smells. It's harder inside the hospital. The doctors and the nurses never experience normal birth ever, because normal birth is when the woman is doing her thing.

The first hands-and-knees birth I ever saw was in midwifery school—a very big, noisy woman was wheeled through the emergency door into the delivery suite. When they went to get her on the table she climbed up onto her hands and knees and there was no moving her. I was with a faculty member who said okay, but the nurses wouldn't come into the room. They walked in and they walked right out. They would not participate with that birth. The woman had a perfectly nice birth, then turned over and picked up her baby, and we rolled her out of there. The nurses did not want to allow her to birth that way—it is an issue of control. That woman is not facing you anymore. You are "en face" with her genitals. The whole hospital is organized to not have that happen except for under very controlled circumstances. It's too sexual.

I was alone in a practice for a year and a half after a midwife had to leave town for two years. It grew up from two or three births a month to seven births a month. I built up my practice through word of mouth. Then I had another midwife join me. But for a year and a half I was on call twenty-four hours a day, seven days a week, and I just went crazy. I missed all the kids' birthday parties. I missed every possible kind of thing like that for years—it was really bad. My partner did try to fill in those gaps when I couldn't be there with the kids. Now my kids both are real proud of my being a midwife. They like that I have this reputation and that people on the street know who I am. They like that I do this kind of work.

After a while I could feel myself going over the edge from the pressure of my practice. It wasn't the births. It was the schizophrenic life of what I did inside that birthing room, under tremendous pressure, and what I had to do on the outside of that door to fend off the community and the nurses. Inside that room I did incredible, creative work to allow and encourage women to be themselves, but that door was like a lid on a pressure cooker. I couldn't function with the staff at the hospital. There was an unbelievable amount of conflict and pressure, and with the lack of support it was very destructive to me. You know the average working life of a certified nurse-midwife is only ten years. And it's not the patients, it's the system. For example, the terribly shoddy physician backup. It is embarrassing to me what I exposed the women to in terms of physician backup, just in order to attend their births. I know

that I did very good work. I know there were a lot of births that were incredibly better because I was there, but I did participate in some way in the institutionalization of the birth center movement. Because I said, "No. We will do it inside and we will do it right here and do it the way we want to. I will do births my own way."

Out of the room I was fending off interference all the time. Hospital personnel could walk in any time they wanted. The doctors are in control, but the nurses are the cops. There was no way you can practice midwifery in that context as far as I was concerned.

After another several months, I was totally whacked. I was under so much pressure that the only thing that was working was my clinical mind and so I didn't kill anybody. But nothing else was working.

So then I announced to the midwifery community that I would give them three months to find me a partner or I'd end the practice. A midwife volunteered to come and cover my practice for a week so that I could take a break and give me some time. When she came I had lost it; I didn't even think that I could come back the next day. There was a woman who came in dilated to seven centimeters, and as I took her into the room the nurse immediately interfered with her. At one point the nurse left the room, and I got a pair of scissors off the table, and I had these scissors in my hand, and I was standing at the door knowing that the next person who walked in the room was getting knifed with these scissors. But it was the other midwife, thank God, so I didn't kill anyone at that hospital. I said to the other midwife, "I'm under too much pressure, I'm out of here." And she said, "Okay, how about you don't come in for two weeks."

Out of that experience she decided to join me. We worked together for three years, and then her husband was offered a tenured job in Ohio, and I said that's it. I had finally experienced a decent partnership and wasn't going to live this lifestyle of a midwife anymore. I tried to practice with several people after that, and I just couldn't get along with anyone.

Later I went to Africa to join this midwifery partner who was working at a birth center in Zimbabwe for three months. We would see 150 women in a morning—they would line up and come in and have their uteruses palpated. I diagnosed six sets of twins in a several-week period. Three-quarters of the women in Zimbabwe still have their babies at home, but this birth center was a central place for women who would come and stay there until they had their baby. We had very little equipment, no oxygen in the tanks that they had, and one bulb syringe for the whole hospital, so if you knew there was meconium

[the baby's first stool; it is sticky and dangerous for the baby to inhale at birth], you'd try to find it. There was no hot running water, and we boiled the reusable syringes. They had one speculum, but they didn't do Pap smears because the labs were unreliable in getting any results.

I spent much time there taking care of the orphans. One of the things I did was to educate the nurses and nurse-midwives about the need for stimulation of newborns, how they don't grow from food alone—they grow from love and being touched. One of the real problems with orphan babies is failure to thrive. They didn't stimulate the babies, but they also didn't believe in adoption in that particular culture. I would ask them to look at the babies. What is this baby trying to tell you? See how he is moving his hands? They just plugged the babies in to bottles and went about their work.

Baby Noah was four or five days old when he came to the clinic. He was his mother's fourth child, and she died a little bit after his birth. I had a passionate love affair with this baby Noah. I even nursed him. This guy was probably eight days old when I went camping for the weekend, and he was thriving and he was doing all right. I was gone for two nights, and when I came back late at night I came into the nursery to see him and he had died. My strong feeling was that he had decided not to do this—twice was enough in being abandoned. At first it felt like I had killed him by offering and then withdrawing. I decided that it was really his decision and that was what he was stuck with. I couldn't have him, they wouldn't allow it, so I think he decided to leave. And when I came back to the United States I looked for him everywhere, I just sensed his presence. Since then every baby that was coming into my life, every baby was maybe him. . . .

He died at the beginning of a long weekend, so they wrapped him up in a swaddling cloth. But they couldn't bury him because they needed someone from his family to come, so they took him to town and put him in a freezer. His father came from way up in the mountains and was a very poor man, but he managed to come to town to sign a release. I met him, and I got someone to translate to him that I had known his baby and what a dear person he was, so I got to have this interaction with this father. The father couldn't stay because he had three more children up in the mountains, so he signed for Noah to be released from the ward and returned to the birth center. The nurses had a ritual that they did around it, they wrapped him in a white box with ribbons and flowers and prepared to bury him in this place where they had buried lots of babies, in a rocky place. A nurse who always did this work said that the mother had to carry the baby and she gave him to me. They

knew that whole time, they knew about my relationship with him. We never talked about it but they knew that he was mine. That was the most intense thing that happened to me in Zimbabwe.

I have diabetes, so it makes it harder to do midwifery and have a life— sometimes I can't do it all. I could never be a full-time midwife again. I abused the diabetes to be able to do midwifery for years. But it isn't okay. Maybe some day I can take care of myself and do midwifery. For now, I like assisting other midwives and not have the responsibility of a full practice.

I think midwifery is revolutionary—that's why it's endangered and dangerous to institutions, because we are one of the few groups of people that believe in the real soul of women and believe that women need independence. And that is very dangerous in our culture because it's not the way our culture or any other culture works. Does it leave me to think we have to have a separatist state? No, I just want us to be in charge. I want women to get an opportunity to run this world—the boys have messed it up. So I feel that midwifery is not only spiritual, it is political.

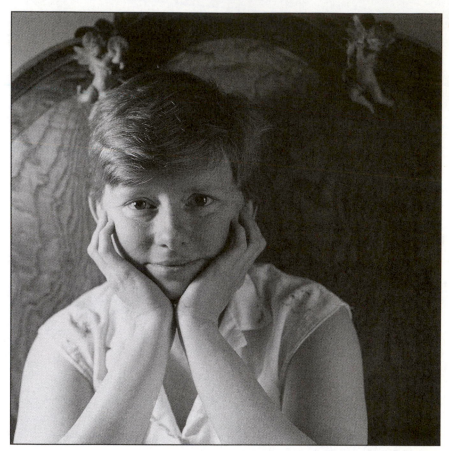

Anne Frye

Anne Frye received a bachelor of arts in holistic midwifery in 1978 and did her clinical birth training at the Maternity Center in El Paso, Texas. She began teaching midwifery intensives through a childbirth education and midwifery organization called Informed Homebirth and has given innumerable workshops all over the country on understanding labwork and suturing skills for midwives. She has authored three books, *Understanding Labwork in the Childbearing Year* (4th ed., 1990), *Healing Passage* (5th ed., 1995), and *Holistic Midwifery. Vol. 1, Care during Pregnancy* (1995). Anne presently lives in Oregon and is the first vice-president of MANA.

Anne Frye

As far back as I can remember I have wanted to be at a birth and have been fascinated with it. It's almost like I've been doing midwifery all my life. The main thing that I played as a child was birth—having babies, catching babies, and being pregnant. And it was definitely the midwifery aspects of having babies, more than having babies to take care of and being a mommy.

When I was young my mother told me about the whole process of birth. I was eight years old when her friend down the street was pregnant. I imagined that no one would be home in the neighborhood when she went into labor and I would be the only one to help her.

Sometimes I thought I'd go to medical school, but I never thought that I could do the chemistry or the math, so I never pursued it. One day I was talking to this cashier in a food co-op who said she was going to be a midwife. Even as she said this I remembered a dream that I had when I was eight or nine, one I hadn't remembered up until that time. It was foggy and at night, and down beside the water on a dock there was a woman in the midst of a crowd who was having a baby. So I helped her. It wasn't a graphic, anatomical dream, but I knew that was what I was doing. So when I remembered that dream I just knew beyond a shadow of a doubt that that was what I was supposed to be—I was going to be a midwife.

I never had any doubt about it after that. Without any thought of what the economic realities of that would be, or anything, I just did it, I pursued it. So I really feel midwifery is my destiny.

I have always said even from the very beginning that I got into midwifery for every spiritual, altruistic, neurotic reason. It meets needs on every level, both functional and dysfunctional for me. Because I can be obsessive-compulsive about my work, midwifery became my whole life. I moved west because I'm looking for a more well rounded situation. Because I feel like midwifery can be a spiritual path. It allows me to be involved with all kinds of people in all walks of life at a very intimate time. It is not a superficial kind of job—it offers me the challenge of being in new situations all the time because each birth is new. When things get too stressful from dealing with on-the-edge situations, I've often joked that I should just be a clerk at Woolworth's, but I could never do that. I get bored too easily. Midwifery affords me enough intellectual challenge and other stimulation to keep me interested. Over the years I have been drawn to different aspects of what our work as midwives entails; it is so multifaceted. Each birth is unique, and it requires you to be a detective, a clinician, and a counselor. It requires so much, and for me that is important.

What I am doing now is working on a textbook for midwives and putting it into three volumes: prenatal, intrapartum, and postpartum. That, with my labwork book and the one on suturing that I have written, will bring my work all together. In working on this it has been great to learn what other midwives have come up with.

A partnership with another midwife in some ways is like a marriage. One of the advantages of working with a partner is to have someone else to bounce ideas and questions off of, someone who has another perspective. We have virtually the same philosophies, spiritual outlooks, and similar clinical background, but I'm very academically oriented and she's very practical and intuitive. When I'm at a birth and have a gut level fear or concern, I always try to check it out with the other midwife, to find out if this is an intuitive sense or just a mental conversation, your mind going on and on that this could be a problem.

My intuition at birth has more to do with tuning in to birthing energy on some subtle level, just allowing myself to be, and paying attention to how I'm feeling as I listen to heart tones or how I'm feeling when I'm palpating a baby. Or how I'm feeling when I meet a woman and how she feels, and her intuitive sense of the baby.

I think that lesbians are unfortunately the unsung heroines of the midwifery movement in the United States. Lesbians have been instrumental in moving nurse-midwifery forward, and for centuries lesbians in general have

been working actively in women's health care. And yet the lesbian issue is a very taboo issue. It is denigrating to feel like you can be here as long as you keep a bag over your head. Therefore, I feel it needs to be spoken about out loud. The more that lesbian midwives feel safe enough to come out and they can identify themselves, it will set the record straight, so to speak.

When people see that the people they work with, and who take care of them at any level—their service people, their medical care providers, their sons and daughters, their aunts and uncles—are the very same people that are lesbians and gays, then it puts it into an entirely different context and makes it harder for lesbians and gays to be the "other weird people."

I feel that we are guardians of women's empowerment through birth. A lot of lesbians see that there is potential empowerment for women on both ends of the spectrum—with family planning and abortion at one end and birth at the other. Not that I think that abortion is any more than a Bandaid on a gushing artery in our culture. Clearly abortion wouldn't be necessary in a system where men totally respected women and women were seen as equal human beings. I think that it is interesting that the Christian Right, which is so totally antiabortion, doesn't understand that the amount of male violence and the rape and the amount of coerced sexual activity that goes on within and outside of marriage is part and parcel of the current cultural need for abortion. And hand-in-hand goes the need for women to respect themselves. You don't get treated like that if you respect yourself.

I have done a lot of work for the midwifery community, and if I had put even half the energy into the lesbian community, I feel that I would have been able to make a difference there too. But the facts are that my destiny is to do that for midwifery. And I am not the only one who is doing that. I work for predominantly heterosexual women—and it is a calling, not a nine-to-five job. So to feel that some of those same women would ostracize or condemn me for who I am is very intense and makes me that much more committed to be out as a lesbian. I made sure I was publicly out before I ran for office in MANA. I chose to come out into the midwifery community after I had made a name for myself with my work as a recognized writer and speaker. Because I thought that with people knowing who I was and then adding to that my being a lesbian would make it harder for them to reject me. And hopefully my coming out would create more safety for other midwives who want to come out. I want to make sure on an organizational level that we don't support the intrinsic homophobia in our culture. Diversity training that we did on the board was so valuable in looking at our oppressive attitudes.

Another part of my organizational work was a call to work on a code of ethics for midwives [see the MANA ethics statement in Appendix A]. At first it was the old "trying to put a square peg in a round hole"—medical ethics don't fit into midwifery values. Because medical ethics are all about power—doctors' authority over patients, policing each other, shepherding the patient through the process—which doesn't have anything to do with what we do. We are basically gounded in an ethic of relationship, in interaction and honesty. Because their ethics don't fit into our values, and values in ethic statements are not stated but are always implicit, I felt like we had to get back to values. So we started with a values statement and then wrote a preamble explaining why our ethics statement primarily consists of a list of values. At the end there is a discussion of how one makes an ethical decision based on one's values, and that's why we can't have an explicit ethics statement because everyone's decisions and how they act is dependent upon their social, cultural, racial, religious, and class background.

Safety is not something I think about very much (any more) because I think safety in birth, for the most part, is medical hype. They have trumped up this idea of safety as being where it's at—I think it is mostly a marketing job. If safety were truly the issue then everybody would be attended at home-births with midwives. It is obvious, the statistics are overwhelmingly in favor of homebirth with midwives. But safety is clearly not the issue—it is self-responsibility.

For example, informed disclosure is a way of exposing myself to my clients and a way of taking on a certain type of accountability. There is really no way a client is going to know how I am going to be in a crisis, but I can tell her what I've seen and how I've conducted myself.

Where I was trained in midwifery, I got this attitude that good midwives don't transport, and that midwives are there to deal with complications. I felt like I was at great odds with my feelings; on one side complications, clinical management, all those kinds of issues, and on the other my intuition and trusting birth. These things were very much at odds within myself. I went to a therapist and sort of cleared up once and for all this conflict between my intuition and being there at births to handle problems, and I realized that I wasn't at births to handle problems; I was there to help the women have the best experience they could have, and with that change in focus, my relationship to birth complications really changed.

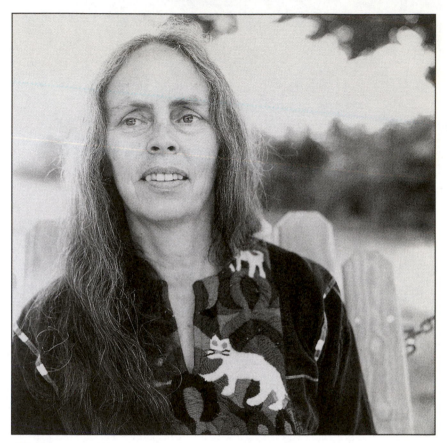

Ina May Gaskin

Ina May Gaskin is a certified professional midwife (CPM) whose original roots in empirical midwifery are documented in the midwifery classic *Spiritual Midwifery*. First published in 1975, this book served as an informal text for lay midwives across the country and included many birth stories. It contains the history of The Farm, an intentional community in rural Tennessee that was formed by a group traveling in a caravan from California. She also wrote *Babies, Breastfeeding and Bonding* (1987) and is the editor of *The Birth Gazette*. Ina May is an internationally known speaker and the current president of MANA. She is the director of The Farm Midwifery Center, a service based at The Farm, whose midwives have attended over eighteen hundred births. Today, with her husband, Stephen Gaskin, they have started a new project called the Rocinante Healing Project, in which health care and community support are offered from "cradle to grave," building birth cottages and cottages for the elderly who want to retire within the context of a supportive community. Ina May is involved with national health care reform and is leading a campaign to articulate and further the midwifery model of care in the United States.

Ina May Gaskin

I came to be a midwife out of a deep feeling in my bones that I knew something about birth, a feeling which arose after hearing women's stories as they told me what birth was like at home. When I went out to California in the late fifties, I met a woman who said that her birth at home didn't hurt anything like it did in the hospital even though she didn't have anesthesia. This woman lived out in the country, and after the baby was born, she looked out the window and the neighbor's cows had walked a quarter mile up the road to look in the window. Now that story got me—I thought, How did the cows know what was going on there? Since then I have found that different species as well as humans gravitate toward birth when the birth feels good to the mother.

What we have in our culture are two very sharply opposed ideas of childbirth. One of them is the traditional Earth Mother—babies fall out of her and she goes back to work; and then you've got birth as probably the most frightening experience awaiting you because it's the worst pain you'll ever feel and if you didn't have a lot of surgery there'd be hell to pay or we'd all be dying. Those are the extremes, and then there are a lot of places in between. I can't tell you the whole story of what happened to me, but it's in my book *Spiritual Midwifery*. Basically, I just started attending births without ever having read anything but one book that was written by an English doctor, Grantly Dick-Reed, called *Childbirth without Fear*. There were no pictures in it, and before I attended my first birth I had never seen a photo-

graph or drawing of birth, which probably seems a little odd to you because they are all over the place now; but really you could be an educated woman in the sixties and any time before that and be curious and go all over to libraries and never see a picture of anything giving birth.

I have never had any formal education in any sort of medical field; I was an English major before I had a child in 1966. I was scared of having a kid in such a dangerous world—I thought it would slow me down if I needed to get away from anything—so I put off having a child till I was out of the Peace Corps, where I first heard of hippies and that gave me hope. The expression of that hope was that I'd get pregnant and have a child.

I know sometimes it sounds like I'm from another planet, but really I'm not, I'm from the Midwest. I was a little bit of an eccentric kid in that I was one of the girls that had a paper route and I was slow at cutting my braids. When I went to junior high I didn't want to get with the program, but I did, and I put my hair in curlers and wore a girdle, so I experienced that side of life too (not that I liked it). I got good grades in school and I liked the boys too. I always wondered about birth and I knew that you had to brave, and I felt that was good because I knew if I was a guy that I would be drafted and people would try to kill me. What did women have to face? We had to face childbirth, and to me that was a sort of testing that represented a coming of age. This younger generation doesn't look at it that way and only wants to be tested in the ways that men are tested.

So my own birth was a big learning experience. I wasn't afraid and was prepared to go in and have the baby without anesthesia—but I had the great surprise that I wasn't allowed to do so. I would have had to get violent and slug the nurse in the delivery room if I didn't want to have spinal anesthesia. So not being trained to be that aggressive and assertive, I had the anesthesia and experienced the results of a subsequent fear that alienated me from myself and made me fearful for the first time of birth. I was actually irrationally afraid of my daughter—at least for her first four years. I'd be in the car with my daughter sitting in my lap, and the window would be half open and I'd have fears that she would somehow get out the window and end up under the car behind me. Weird stuff.

So when I started to attend births I treated women the opposite way that I'd been treated, and guess what happened? We had 187 babies before we ever had a C-section. Now that's strange isn't it? If the medical field has it right about childbirth, then it shouldn't happen that an English major would just start out to be a midwife not even knowing such a thing existed in this

whole country—and just start doing it with this group of friends and end up with the success that we had. Something was not scientific here. I had some scientific training, and with the national C-sec rate what it was, and because you were American, it was expected that we were going to run into a lot of CPD [cephalo-pelvic disproportion—where the baby's head is too big to come through the mother's pelvis during the birth process]. It wasn't until I sat down at the computer three years ago and put the statistics together for the 1,780 births we had attended that I saw how striking this was. Now these weren't women who were selected to have a big pelvis; this was just the random person who ended up with us. And why did they have the ability to give birth without anesthesia?

I think it was because of the group experience. The first birth that I attended was for a woman who was so happy to be on her bed that she didn't care if it was in a school bus in a parking lot at Northwestern with me who had never seen a birth before. She was happier to see me than she would have been to see either of the two doctors that attended her other births. She had the baby in about two hours, and she looked gorgeous. Nobody had ever told me that women in labor could look beautiful. I couldn't quit looking at her, and because I was looking at her in an appreciative way, she worked better and so I couldn't have told you if she was in pain. She wouldn't have told you she was being brave. She would have told you she was being a coward—brave would have been to go back to the hospital with the way the hospital was in those days. When she had the baby, as a group we felt the energy.

We were a group of four hundred people traveling across the country in the fall and winter of 1970–1971 in school buses we had made into campers. We were on a speaking tour, and that's how these babies were happening on university campuses and national parks and on the main streets of little towns. When people had the experience of this first woman giving birth so easily, it made the birth easier for the next woman, because she thought, Well, if Anna can do that, I think I could. Any fears we may have gotten from our own mothers or girlfriends who had already given birth weren't amplified by the media the way it is now because childbirth didn't really appear in literature or in the movies very much. I had an hour instruction in emergency childbirth by a doctor while we passed through Rhode Island. By the fourth birth we had some problems, we had a hemorrhage and we had to resuscitate the baby. But anybody who wasn't right there didn't know that there were any problems, and they were comparatively easy to solve—give the baby a breath, give the mom a shot of oxytocin [a synthetic hormone that stimulates con-

tractions to control bleeding] and the hemorrhage stops. It was all pretty straightforward, and we sailed through things like that.

When we settled in Tennessee we were too big of a group for any hospital to say, "Come on in—you don't have any money and you have twenty-five pregnant women." There is no licensing of lay midwives in Tennessee, so they gave me birth certificates, death certificates, and ampules of silver nitrate [used to prevent infection in a newborn's eyes], and I understood that what I was supposed to do was to tell the truth on the birth certificate, and I can tell you we have done that for twenty-two years. We have never fudged a number. Unfortunately, with some independent midwives who are in states where they are illegal or have rules and regs that constrict them, they fudge their statistics. For example there are women in Florida, where there are rules that do not allow midwives to attend women at home after their fifth pregnancy, who are having their third baby three or four times according to the state's records. Now this does not get us anywhere—information from birth certificates then is not real or useful.

The prenatal care we do is more than the weighing and measuring that gets put on the chart. Prenatal care is finding out if the mom's scared, what she thinks about childbirth, and cluing her in to where she feels a sense of power about it. With childbirth there is pain, but with birth pain can come ecstasy if the people that are with you take the trouble to treat you like a goddess, and that's the way we think women should go through childbirth. My own feeling is that if you don't go through what nature has laid out for you that you don't fully access that power. The pain of labor is bearable unless women have too much fear about childbirth. I *want* to see the epidural rate go down. I think its nice that we have epidurals [regional anesthesia used to deaden the sensation of contractions during labor or surgery] for when they are truly necessary, but something's wrong when we have women more scared about childbirth now than they were when they had a higher chance of dying.

What I do is joke with women and try to prepare them by saying, "Bring your sense of humor when you have the baby. We want to make you laugh because then it won't hurt as much. Then you'll be telling jokes because you want to laugh." And I'm talking about the belly laughs—a hearty laugh is the best anesthesia of all. We tell stories that connect her to her power.

I've had a lot of hours at labors to think about how our culture thinks about birth, and I think it's because men decide how childbirth will be done.

Men's ideas have formed the whole structure and the knowledge that's available to most people—we don't have a clue about birth because men are totally confused about women's bodies because we are so different from them. And then there is this whole convenience that if women think their bodies don't work then you can make a lot of money inventing gadgets and all sorts of medications. So there is a powerful economic element there too—that's almost bigger than we can imagine.

I publish a magazine, *The Birth Gazette,* in which I have interviews with all the different women that inspire me to let people know that midwives are out there. It's hard to be the kind of midwife I am and not be poor. I'm doing it because I'm trying to keep the door open, and so if I'm to make a living at it, I have to write too.

I don't have and couldn't afford malpractice insurance—there are no companies yet that would give it to a midwife that is not a certified nurse-midwife. I have a different kind of certification that we developed over the years that is rigorous, but it's new enough that the insurance companies don't yet cover us all, although there's one that is looking at doing it now. So how do I protect myself? I don't advertise on a billboard that says, "You will have guaranteed a perfect, safe lovely birth if you go to Ina May." But you see that with the marketing of hospitals—promises are made that can't be kept, and I think that this generation of birthing women is being led to believe anything is possible with modern medicine and technology and it isn't. We're not even doing as well as we could be in this country because we leave so many out of care—we have second-class care for poor people, and wealthier women who have insurance get care that messes up their births. Both of those situations lead us to having one of the highest infant mortality rates in the industrialized world, and we're not doing anything about it. In fact, it's getting worse. So, we've got problems that we have to fix.

Now at long last we have health care reform in this country, and we midwives had better make sure we are a part of it or we will surely be left out. As midwives in rural Tennessee, we were the first people and sometimes the only people that those in the neighboring community would have as primary health care givers. Even though we would primarily be for childbearing women, we would often see all members of the family because they had little contact with other caregivers. There was a country doctor who came and schooled us, not only in birth, but in primary health care. He said, "You have to learn country medicine. There is no way I can take on all your people and all the Amish and these rural Tennesseans." We are one of the vast rural areas

that is medically underserved, and it's even worse now than it was twenty years ago. So for a hundred dollars a week he'd come out to our community and check out the women we needed him to for the things that we couldn't figure out. He taught us how to deal with ear infections, listen to lungs, and saw that we were fast learners.

About ten years ago he said that the Amish practice was too much for him, his practice was growing and he couldn't lure people in to do rural medicine, so he told the Amish elders that they were going to have to accept us as their care providers. The Amish community also have their own grandmothers who serve at their grandchildren's births. And some of these women have had twelve babies themselves, so they know a fair amount about deliveries, but when it gets out of the ordinary where they used to call the doctor, they call us instead. Now we are training three or four midwives in that community.

I've seen my neighbors lose their homes and grow destitute because one person had a serious illness such as diabetes. So I try to look at health care in its simplest equation. What do you need for health care? You need people who need care, people who give care, and people to keep some records and keep track of how this care is paid for. You don't need as many people keeping track as you do people giving care.

Now I pushed very hard and was able to go to a meeting at the White House as part of the group that was reviewing the Clinton health plan as it was being evolved. I was there with rural practitioners, most of them family practice doctors. We were told after a long description of the plan that the rural areas will suffer greatly during the time of reform, which may take as long as two or three decades. It's going to be based upon huge purchasing alliances that will compete with each other, and the theory is that this will lower the cost of health care. Now, in the rural areas we know that things don't work like this and that in any case there will be no competition in the rural areas—we'll be lucky if we have caregivers at all. I say this because I want you to remember rural areas in the United States involve about half of all people.

When it comes to formulating law, rural midwives are at a great disadvantage. This is because the rural midwife is usually very busy—her phone is ringing off the wall, she spends hours and hours with women, and she has little time for political organization. She is also out in the countryside, and she is separated from knowing what is going on, [unlike in places] where midwives find it easier to get together and meet.

Historically, the law has not been used to promote mother and child health as it relates to midwifery. We must realize that. That's what people tend to think, but the reverse is true. The law regarding midwifery in most states in the United States has worked directly against the health of mothers and babies. It has protected the turf of the people who receive money for taking care of mothers and babies. And only for the ones they consent to take care of—the rest are left to fend for themselves; they're invisible to the system. Infant mortality rates are shockingly high in this country—they're worse if we are talking about African American babies, or even worse if we're talking about native American babies. These rates are going up, and the differential between the white babies and the African American babies is getting worse as we sit here. How many of you know that the maternal mortality rate is rising?

I'd say most women of color who are midwives are probably working in birth centers or hospitals or neighborhood clinics, but there are also quite a few in the Muslim community who do homebirths, and there are native American women who work on reservations and Latino women who work in their communities. I'm really glad to see that this movement has spread out over all different cultural groups.

I think that midwives can be peacemakers and community builders, not just in rural areas, but in the most crowded of cities and the poorest circumstances. We do not have a chance of doing this, however, if we keep the costs at current levels for educating midwives. Right now nurse-midwifery education usually involves fifty thousand to one hundred thousand dollars, and when midwives come out of it in such debt it keeps the midwives out of the neighborhoods that most need them. We have to remove the barrier of having to enter the profession of nursing to get to midwifery.

In our community, although we had never read anything about this, it was the midwives that naturally gravitated toward being with families who were dealing with death. Everyone noticed that death felt much like birth, that there was the same sort of energy—a very heightened awareness. Things and people looked dear to you; you had the sense of life being precious, of the need to be good to each other, of the need to be thankful for life, of the need to be attentive to what you had to say, of the need to mix sadness and laughter, to tell stories, to come together and to be very human with each other. Not to think about money, not to think about what would anybody think.

My own baby was the first one in our community that died. I was in the first few months of my midwifery practice, exhausted and anemic, and he was born very premature and lived for twelve hours. I knew that he couldn't have

been saved at that time, so we didn't go to the hospital. We did what we could, but I knew from losing him, I learned a lot. I think if it had happened to somebody else I wouldn't be a midwife now. But because I had the support of the community, I learned about grieving. I also knew that in some way that happened to teach me something important as a midwife and so I tell that story. I've learned about healing, and I learned about how you treat somebody who has lost her baby and about that hunger that women have when they've lost a baby. I understand those women that you hear about in the news who go into the maternity ward and dress up as a nurse to steal somebody's baby. There's a real raw hunger that develops. And women who lose a baby (and this affects the population explosion too) want two more to replace that one. That's why I had three kids after that.

We can't avoid all tragedy; we can't take all the pain out of life because then there's no joy there either 'cause you're just not feeling anything then. The family, or people who are close to the person who is in the passage of being born or who is leaving, need to have what I would call sacred space. They need to be protected from insensitive people, from intrusions by people who don't know what is going on. They need to have their needs seen to, even if they are not able to articulate them themselves. I think that it is no coincidence that in most communities around the world and in all times those people have been midwives. Midwives are a kind of gatekeeper—the energy of birth is much like the energy that surrounds death. Sacred space isn't so much physical space, although it may be, it's the emotional and spiritual space. It means that somebody's there to deal with someone when the meter reader turns up and he's got to do what he needs to do, and she answers the phone, and finds the kids a place to play.

A labor can take a long time; someone needs to think what we may need to eat three hours from now. The same thing happens when there is grief around. People aren't anchored that strongly in their own physical body to feel that they're hungry; they lose their appetite unless someone is seeing to that, and that's why people who are grieving often get sick.

We have to get over being afraid of tears and being afraid to talk about the person who dies. You've got to be able to sit there and listen, and when you hear those stories, if you've got any fear of death yourself, it's going to come up. But you are going to receive something if you sit there and listen. It's not good to carry around a huge load of fear about something that you are guaranteed going to for certain pass through. We are all going to die.

Several years ago I found out that my nineteen-year-old daughter had a

terminal illness. It was the hardest of all the deaths that I had to face. Before she died I got to take her to Wales to our family burial ground. To keep up our spirits we listened to songs of struggle from South Africa as we traveled— and when we got there we read on a tombstone: "It is well to contemplate death."

Death at home is just as important as birth at home and is something that midwives can help out with. Some of the things that are craziest about our culture is that we have become so afraid of both that we don't know how to live. Both my dad and my daughter died at home, and I was with both of them. My dad chose to leave privately, that was kind of what he was like. Our whole clan had gathered together; all my sisters and grandkids were in the house, so there was noise, and life went on, and I know my dad loved that. He had everybody that had come after him in that house, dealing with what- ever we had to deal but mostly just enjoying being together. That was a sense of a life well lived.

When my daughter passed she wanted us with her, and when it came her time she gradually declined. She packed all of what her life could be in eighty years into twenty years, and she could accept that—and because she could I could. We were all holding each other and I felt just a moment of fear in there. I told her it was all right, she could let go. She went out with this look of wonder—just like a kid diving the first time into something new, just like a newborn. One of the most amazing things I've seen. If you don't re- claim these passages and allow them to take place in the home, you don't really fully experience them. We could get a lot saner if we could learn how to accept death, and how to make it a part of life.

My husband and I have a new project; we bought the hundred acres next to The Farm and we are calling it the Rocinante Healing Project. We plan to make cottages for people who at retirement time want to be with people in a community that they know and love while it is their time to go out. When they die that place will be there for someone else to move into. We want to have a birth center too, and we'll have the whole circle. We want to have ten birthing cottages, a midwifery school, and a video studio to make birth videos. I want to see people giving birth on television, tell stories about death at home, so we become more compassionate as a people. I'm con- vinced that if we make a nice place for babies to land, it will be a nice place for the rest of us.

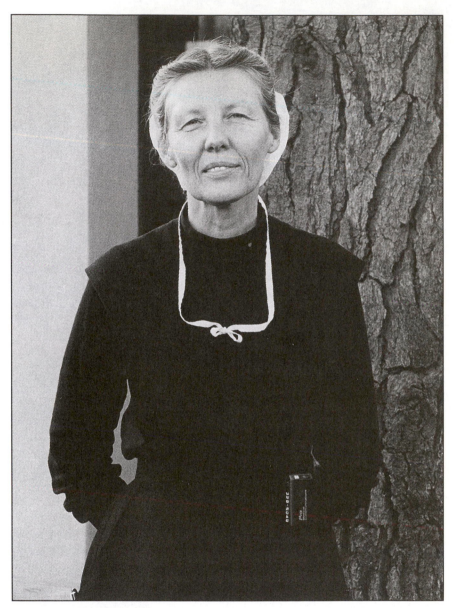

Faith Gibson

Faith Gibson is a domiciliary midwife and administrator of the Mennonite Order of Maternal Services. She lives in Palo Alto, California. The mother of three adult children, she has been attending to the needs of mothers and babies since 1961 in different capacities. In 1991 she was arrested for a number of criminal charges related to practicing midwifery, charges that were eventually dropped when legal research established that traditional or nonmedical midwifery was not a criminal offense in California. Faith did most of the legal research for her own case. She continues to attend births of those parents who consider their choice to birth at home a religious decision. Faith is also a certified hang glider pilot, dulcimer musician, and Scottish country dancer.

Faith Gibson

I was a labor and delivery nurse for a very long time, fifteen years or so, and I left it because I felt that I was continually required to do medical procedures that I knew were not in the best interest of mothers and babies, and that in some instances were even dangerous. There were occasional circumstances in my work as a delivery room nurse in which mothers or babies died as a result of the care that our hospital considered to be the typical standard, which was: Don't ask questions, just do what you're told; such as medicating mothers who were nine centimeters and pushing with high doses of IV narcotics. Then the babies didn't breathe and had to be resuscitated. Then they sometimes blew out the babies' lungs, causing a pneumothorax [the result of air escaping through the injured lung into the cavity outside the lung] which can sometimes be fatal, when they were trying to resuscitate, and so on and so forth.

So I left maternity nursing and joined a domestic Peace Corps project, a VISTA project, in North Carolina. At the end of my assignment I was informally reassigned to work at the San Francisco International Airport with the Vietnamese boat people. This was the late seventies, early eighties. I originally came to California with absolutely nothing; I moved my family myself and I was divorced at that time. It was my intention to never see another pregnant woman as long as I lived if I could help it. I felt what nowadays we would call burnout in terms of hospital nursing. I cannot remember how I got involved with the midwifery community here in the state of California.

I had been doing political organizing work with the domestic Peace Corps project. I did what was called community development, where you go out into the community and meet with the people at churches to identify a need the community had, then you'd work to identify the first necessary steps to take, and finally bring your ideas to the attention of whomever it needs to be brought to. So as a result of the community organizing I was doing, I wound up working with Jerry Brown (who was governor of California) and his administration, which, at least on the surface and in theory, was very alternative medicine–friendly. I've seen some documents since then that make me think that he was not, that the administration overall was not as friendly to alternative medicine as they were making themselves out to be. Either that or the right hand knoweth not what the left was doing.

But in any case, one of the "alternatives" was midwifery, and there was in California a midwifery advisory council, kind of like the dairy advisory council in dairy-farming states and the citrus advisory council, and so on and so forth. It is usually nongovernment people, people who are involved in whatever that industry or occupation is, who meet with the state officials and try to figure out how the state can help you to achieve your goal. Economic solvency, stuff like that. So I worked with this midwifery advisory council as a media person, and we met with then-governor Brown on one of the occasions when we were there in Sacramento working with midwifery legislation. He said, "What you guys need is some media that tells people about midwifery, particularly state senators." And I said, "I'll write the script," and someone else said, "Well, I have some pictures." It turned out the other person was a practicing midwife who lived in Palo Alto, which is about thirty-two miles south of San Francisco, where I was living at the time. So I wound up moving to Palo Alto. I worked with her for maybe six months, and then her partner quit practicing, and I apprenticed with her.

It was interesting, because I thought I was doing her a big favor, because after all, I had been a labor and delivery room nurse. I would know what to do when someone's uterus ruptured, or when the babies didn't breathe, which was the only kind of maternity care I'd ever seen—ones in which you assumed that a lot of the babies would not breathe, because after all the mothers were anesthetized, or they were narcotized, or both. This was in the early eighties, before the hospitals got on the bandwagon of alternatives. The only choices were highly medicalized births which didn't permit husbands to be present, or homebirths. And in some ways that made the choices easier, because people just split down the middle. So after the first

fifty births, after I had worked with her for about a year, I finally went, "Well, what is wrong with this picture? How come I'm not getting to run around and do emergency maternity nursing?"

Then I started to examine more the principles that are involved in midwifery. Before that I didn't really think that homebirth was better or safer— other than obviously it was cheaper. So after the first fifty births I really started wondering how come these people aren't having complications? I thought birth was complex. That was the reason we had all those complications in a medical setting; those people were lucky to be there. They just happened to be in the right place at the right time. I *did* see the association between things like giving Demerol and scopolamine [a sedative that produces amnesia] to multips [women who had given birth before] who were nine centimeters, and then rupturing their membranes. I could see how that resulted in a baby with respiratory distress, but I didn't see the obstructions of labor, the funky psychological obstructions of labor. I just didn't appreciate what I now recognize as the traditions of midwifery and the fundamental soundness of the principles of midwifery until after I had been really quite exposed to it. I don't know, it's like something changed in my brain, and I couldn't go back to the "other way." Even when I left nursing in 1976, I had in my mind the conversation about war crimes during the Second World War—people who ran concentration camps and did medical experiments called into account when the war was over, and it wasn't sufficient to say, "My commanding officer told me to, sir!" The people said *you're* responsible for what you do, even if somebody else tells you to do it. If you carried it out, you did it. I went, what's the difference? I'm a labor and delivery room nurse, and somebody says, "Give this lady a hundred of Demerol," this tiny, little, petite woman who's nine centimeters and beginning to push. It's my job to do—I was fired a lot, I have to tell you. My nursing career was kind of a rocky course.

One of the early times that I was fired, I talked to the doctor who was chief of ob/gyn for that year—he was really a nice man—and he said, "Honey, if the doctor orders strychnine, you either give strychnine, or *you chart* that you gave strychnine." That's a direct quote. This would have been about 1965. The idea was that you did what you were told, that was what your job was—the job of the nurse was to carry out the physician's orders. It was not your job to think, to ask questions. I couldn't keep doing that.

I'm not against medical care when it's for a clear and present need. I'm against the kind of medical care that's being done either out of habit, eco-

nomic advantage to the care provider, or cost shifting, risk shifting, and blame shifting.

The hospital that I trained in and worked in was segregated. That means that the black mothers were admitted to the postpartum beds rather than to the labor room, because the labor room was all white. So the postpartum bed was one in a four-bedroom ward. The other woman could be having her gall bladder out, or be a diabetic with an infected foot. They tried not to mix infection with noninfected circumstances, but you know how hospitals are, you can't always achieve your goals there.

So I saw those black mothers come in, and they were not medicated because there wasn't anyone to watch them. You can't give scopolamine to somebody unless there's an attendant constantly present to keep that person from falling out of bed. And another reason for not medicating them was the idea that black mothers were sort of primitive, like a subspecies that weren't like us post–Queen Victoria white ladies. We were all sort of tied up in knots and we fainted a lot, and we couldn't get it together. We needed a lot of help. Whereas, the reasoning went, black mothers were more like farm animals, and they just drop the kids out. Also, they were really, typically, higher parity [having had a greater number of births], and when you're dealing with really high parity, they really do drop their babies out like that.

So without medication when they got ready to have the baby, you could tell because you could hear her making sounds. We would go get a stretcher and drag her off of her bed, on to the stretcher, go peeling off down the hall, get in the elevator, go up five floors, and then go down another hall into the delivery rooms upstairs. They could deliver in the delivery rooms upstairs, but they couldn't labor in the labor rooms, because that was white only.

In reality what happened was that we delivered them in that elevator between the first and the fifth floor. We just flipped the switch off so that it wouldn't open up when you'd be in the middle of having a baby, and there would be this whole crowd going, "Oh, that's kind of interesting." It wasn't so much that we were taking authority of some sort as that it was a modesty issue. It was just considered to be rude to have them be so exposed.

Simultaneously, upstairs, where the white women were admitted, the first thing that they did was the traditional prep and enema, and then they gave them a double dose of sleeping pills. Then somewhere around three or four centimeters' dilation they started to give them a hundred milligrams of Demerol with scopolamine and morphine or viosterol [a sedative-hypnotic

drug]. These women would drool, they were so out of it. Then when they finally became completely dilated, we took them to the delivery room and put them in stirrups and sprayed their genitals with mercurochrome and draped them and got them all ready for the doctor, who came along and promptly did a great big episiotomy and then a low forceps delivery. The mother was then sent off, still unconscious, to recover, and the baby, whom she's never laid eyes on, was sent off to the nursery, and sometime in the next twelve hours if they were lucky, they got to wave at each other. That was normal birth.

And simultaneously these black women had their babies in the elevator. It's like, what is wrong with this picture? So I never believed that birth was not a normal process, but I simultaneously believed in the capacity for it to go awry. I didn't see an association between hospitalization and medicalization and intervention as the source of those problems. I saw it only from the standpoint—and this is typical, I think—that labor and delivery room nurses and obstetricians today reflect exactly this same opinion, which is one of the reasons I have so much respect for what it is we need to do as midwives. Because I shared that opinion that childbirth was complex and dangerous.

I remember when the midwife I trained with told me that she was going to do a homebirth for a woman whose last baby was born by cesarean. My mouth fell open. I remembered people having ruptured uteruses, somebody running to hold the elevator while this team of people pulled the stretcher, and they're all barreling down, and we were hoping to get the arteries to her uterus tied off before she bled to death. The idea that this woman was going to do a homebirth for someone who'd had a cesarean—this was long before there was a vocabulary for any of this—I thought she was crazy. I didn't call the police and report her, but it ran through my mind. Not quite that, but I really thought she had taken leave of her senses in a really big, heavy-duty, for-real way. Then I eventually started providing labor support for VBAC [vaginal birth after cesarean] mothers. I did all this hospital VBAC stuff. I noticed that as long as they had no other problems than VBAC status, everyone worried about the previous cesarean scar. If the labor was slow, membranes were ruptured for more than twenty-four hours, heart tones were this, that or the other thing, we only talked about those things, we never talked about their VBAC status. But if they were normal and they didn't have something wrong with their labor or their baby, then we did all this, "Of course, she's a VBAC, na-na-na."

I eventually wound up doing VBACs myself as a midwife, and I remem-

ber one of the nurse-midwives in the area, whom I greatly admired—if anyone could be called a really good Christian lady, this is the woman—who was
horrified that I was doing VBACs, because I was going to bring not only
disaster on the mothers and babies that I dealt with, but on the nurse-midwives. Midwifery in general was going to suffer because I was going out on
this limb and doing VBACs. Well, now, *she* does VBACs at home.

But the assumption was made by both myself and what one would nowadays call a preceptor or mentor that I knew what I was doing, and so the
senior midwife went to Mexico and said, "I'm going for a month, this lady's
due . . . and this lady . . . and this lady." I was a midwife—kind of like that
joke, last week I couldn't spell it and now I am one. I didn't set out to be a
midwife. I really didn't.

I suffered, I really did, in terms of the psychological guilt that came from
my years of obstetrical nursing. I didn't want anything to do with the unhappi-
ness that had come about for me in that work even though maternity nursing is
supposed to be happy work. But nurses do a lot of arguing, backbiting—it's
weird, any time you're in such a powerless position, you tend to turn around
and use what little bit of power you have against people under you.

In fact, my lawyer once made a comment that you either take orders or
you take risks. Midwives take risks, and nurses take orders. And part of taking
orders is that you always are looking for somebody that you can boss around
and you can turn around and pass it on. So there was all this grief, and a lot of
the grief had to do with the quality of these unnecessary interventions, with
things that were invasive and unpleasant and dangerous.

I remember in 1974, there was an article that was published by Niles
Newton on pubic preps. They had done a retrospective, a controlled study. I
don't remember the specifics of it, but the prepped women had more infections than the unprepped women. So I put that up on the wall over the urinal
in the doctors' lounge. It didn't make any difference. Nothing made any
difference. They did what they did and that was it. They harassed me, and one
doctor actually accused me of being a witch because my patients did so well.
Why all this grief? I finally decided to leave.

I have been innately a religious or spiritual person. I don't know why,
but it just seems like that's always been a large part of my psyche. As a student
nurse I was trained in nursing by a woman who taught nursing as a religious
vocation, who went into nursing in the late 1920s. This was a time when if
you chose to be a nurse you chose not to get married, you chose not to be a
mother. It was an either/or decision.

I think I was just born to be a midwife. I found my niche, but what I'm saying is I didn't seek it out. I didn't start out with the theoretical concept like perhaps many young women who are going into midwifery today. They have the concepts about midwifery, and then they get the rude shock, the reality. Because you have to get up in the middle of the night, and you don't get to go home when you're tired and want to sleep, and your kids need you, and it's your birthday or it's Christmas. I've had a fair number of apprentices who were very interested in the concepts of midwifery, but you couldn't wake them up in the middle of the night. They'd go, "I can't come. I have to do something in the morning." I'd go, "You don't really have a choice. I'm going to be there in fifteen minutes and you'd better have your britches on." After a while they were no longer an apprentice.

So when I found myself managing these homebirths for my midwife mentor who went to Mexico for a month, it was like I was suddenly an adult for the first time. I was making the decisions that needed to be made and doing the things that needed to be done, and the babies were coming out. They breathed. Nobody's uterus was rupturing. Well, we weren't giving pitocin to these people. No wonder their uteruses weren't rupturing. Why didn't we ever connect that up?

There's another strong element in me—I've probably participated in about thirty-five hundred hospital births. That means that for a fair number of those women I did pubic preps, soapsuds enemas, medicated them with barbiturates and narcotics. Babies died as a result of that. I can remember babies that died of patients I cared for. No one is going to legally pursue me for that, but I know that I did that. I was involved in a birth in which the mother died, and I know that it was as a result of criminal behavior on the part of the physician, truly criminal behavior. It was the woman's second baby, so she left two motherless little kids. She died not because she was unhealthy or her pregnancy was abnormal or there was an earthquake and no medical care was available. She died because her doctor was going someplace and he wanted to get her delivered so he could leave town. He did things that resulted in an amniotic fluid embolism [sudden blocking of an artery due to amniotic fluid entering the bloodstream], and she died, just like that. A gush, a huge quantity of blood, and the baby's father had just left the delivery room with the baby when she left the planet. As a nurse, "carrying out doctor's orders," I did a lot of stuff, and I guess I just had to karmically make up for it.

When I was being prosecuted for practicing midwifery, people always said to me, "Why don't you just become a nurse-midwife?" And I'd become

totally inarticulate. Why *don't* I just become a nurse-midwife? That story was so intense that I couldn't tell it, couldn't communicate. I just wanted to shoot them, strangle them. What it means to get through nurse-midwifery school is to be willing to be a little bit untruthful with your clients and a little bit unkind, and in fact sometimes a little bit cruel.

You deliver twenty babies as a student nurse-midwife. Five of them have to have episiotomies, because that's what the rules are in order for you to graduate. It's not based on whether the mother needed an episiotomy. It's based on the fact that the midwife needed the experience. That's like having student surgeons shoot people in the foot so they can practice getting those bullets out and sewing up the holes afterward. That's why I'm not going to become a nurse-midwife, or a licensed midwife under the new California bill. It's an unworkable bill. No one else will become a licensed midwife under it either except people who are already trained through nurse-midwifery. It's identical to nurse-midwifery. A nurse-midwife could become a licensed midwife without doing anything different, but for those of us who are traditional midwives, it's not going to work.

I am fortunate enough to practice under the religious exemption clause at a time in history when it's almost unheard of and poorly understood. That means that I have the privilege of providing nonmedical, nonsurgical care to families who are asking for care under the religious exemption clause, who have in essence made the decision for themselves, speaking of informed choice, to have a nonmedical birth in their own home, and they are seeking out an experienced helper to assist them in the choice that they've made. They have to sign papers—request for care under the religious exemption clause. To a large extent I work with people who are uniquely suited to the choice they've made. They are rarely people whose religious belief structure prevents medical care in an emergency. They're making the distinction that childbirth is not an emergency, that childbirth is normal life, and in normal life we normally use social structures of support rather than medical, and that social support structure includes things such as prayer.

When I talk about prayer, I'm talking about listening as well as talking. A lot of people think about prayer as you sit down and tell God what to do now, give Him a little list of what you want, and that it's something that one does fairly rarely, like pray on Sunday morning for the rest of the week. Whereas I would think of prayer as listening, as a constant saying, basically, is there anything here I need to know that I don't know? Is there something we need to do that we're not doing? Give me a little clue if there is. For instance,

the mother's water breaks and tons of meconium [the baby's first stool; it is sticky and dangerous for the baby to inhale at birth] come out, and I go, "Got it. We're going to the hospital." The male, linear mode is an either/or mode: you either have a highly medicalized hospital birth, or you have an unattended birth. That's the medical model. They don't see a middle ground between those two things. So the people I work with represent that middle ground. They are (a) committed to having a normal, natural birth in a non-medical setting and (b) receptive to the possibility that they will need medicalization, that if a true emergency arises, I am going to say something equivalent to, "I'm going to the hospital, I hope you'll join me. I'm going to get the car now and pull it right up here, and I'm going to put my bags in it. I hope . . ." and they come with me. I've never had anyone actually, completely refuse hospital care when I felt it was necessary.

It is that the parent herself must define the choice as religiously based. I think that we have an ethical responsibility to our children that cannot be turned over to the institutions of modern society. We can enlist the assistance of the institutions of modern society in achieving the goals that we've identified as necessary or desirable, but we can't give over to the institutions of society everything, the care, the decision-making process. So people need to be willing to state that at a level that were we to go to court and they would be sworn in, they would be able to say, "Yes, I signed this document. And it was true."

So that means that sometimes I lose families that liked me personally, but couldn't bring themselves to see what they're doing as religious. And that's actually okay, because I do think about it as a three-way activity going on between myself and the family that I'm working with and whatever you want to call the higher power. In other words, I'm not taking responsibility alone. I'm saying, "Look, you and I together with God are going to do our best job. That's the best I can tell you."

That's a very large chunk of what shows up culturally as the malpractice crisis, because we go to this person and say, "Here, you make all the decisions, and if you're wrong I'm going to sue you." And I'm saying, "I'm not making those decisions for you. You and I together with God make those decisions, but I'm not making them for you."

A lot of people, they don't get it. They want somebody who will tell them what they need to do. And I think that those kind of people really are best served by people who are state-certified, who have that whole web of structure around what they do. What happens is they just pass it around. You

go to this person, and he says, "Oh, well, you should have an ultrasound." And the ultrasound person says, "Oh, well, you need a biophysical profile." Pretty soon you get fifteen people involved in this, none of whom are personally responsible, including the mother and father.

I've seen a lot of life. That's one of the things about being an emergency nurse, you see a lot of things that you wouldn't otherwise be exposed to, and I kind of had a sense of myself as pretty well rounded and well experienced. But I had never experienced some of the things that went along with being arrested and prosecuted. One of the things is that 90 percent of the people I thought I could count on were useless. They didn't know what to do, to say; they said things like, "Why don't you just become a nurse-midwife? It's your fault. You just do what you're supposed to, you wouldn't be in this problem."

And that included the midwifery organizations. If you were a physician being prosecuted in the way that I was, the California Medical Association would be right there with you. They'd hire lawyers, it'd be a big deal. Well, the California Midwives' Association does not do that. Partly, obviously, because of the economics of it all. But the fact that 90 percent of the people I knew did not come through was really shocking. That's the only word for it.

However, a lot of people I didn't know or would have never thought to count on, or to think of in that way, came through. So I often think and talk about it as a whole bunch of new friends, a different set of friends. In some ways it's like I have something in my gut in having been down right to the bottom line of something that gives you a certain kind of confidence, that you know something of your abilities that you didn't know before. Of course, at this point in time, I've gone completely through a circle. There's an insight or peacefulness that wasn't present before the circle was concluded. I didn't know how it was going to come out before it came out, until they dropped the charges.

I had been charged with everything—the oil spill in the Gulf, practically everything in the world. I was charged with practicing medicine without a license, nursing, midwifery, nurse-midwifery, advertising without a license. I had five charges against me. That's a tactic of intimidation. They charge you with everything in the world, knowing that you're going to have to pay thousands of dollars to pay a lawyer to go through these charges one by one. There's no sense to them, but you don't know that, and your lawyer certainly isn't going to tell you that there's no substance to these charges. The lawyer's going to tell you about how much you need him. That kind of thing.

Dealing with lawyers was probably the most distressing, short of the reality of being arrested and having people come to your door, put handcuffs on you, and take you away in front of your minor children, which was what happened. Dealing with lawyers was like dealing with obstetricians. There's a whole agenda there that has nothing to do with my particular circumstance or the ethics of my case or any of those kinds of things. Lawyers have the same kinds of constraints on them that obstetricians do, which is that if they don't do what they are supposed to do they face being ostracized by their fellow lawyers and, more specifically, threats of being disbarred by the judges if they say things the judge doesn't like. It's like an obstetrician is always working to make sure he doesn't lose his hospital privileges, a lawyer is always working to make sure he doesn't lose his lawyer privileges.

I believe there's been a fundamental error on the part of midwives as a class and on the part of individual midwives who have been prosecuted, in that we went to lawyers and said, "Tell us what to do." This is like going to your obstetrician and saying, "What should I do?" What can either a lawyer or an obstetrician say but the most conservative advice, the thing that is the best for him in terms of economic outcome and least risky? Well, what midwives need to do is to follow the actual research on medical practice and continue to research the application of the midwifery tradition. We need to go to lawyers and say, "This is what we want you to do now. We're hiring you to achieve these goals. Here's the information, here's what we want to do with it, and here's what we want you to do. You want the job? Well, this is what you've got to do." Midwives have not done that. They've gone to lawyers and they've said, "Oh, help us." Lawyers are not God. We went to lawyers as if they were, and they aren't. I guess maybe one shouldn't be so surprised that the outcome of my case was less than the best. Particularly in California, I don't know about other states, but you look at the actual records of California and you will see what the state has done to midwives there. One of these days they'll do a major TV miniseries. It's too long for a made-for-TV movie, because they've been doing this for a long time.

The two best things to come out of my court case were—one is that we have a court document that verifies the religious exemption clause, confirms the legality of religious exemptions in the practice of midwifery, and the second thing is the legal research that I did. I like doing that kind of research. I'm a good scholar. I like to go to the library, see all those books. I'd go to the stacks at Stanford Library and go, "Ahhhh." The frustration has been that the midwifery community, because they were involved in this legislative pur-

suit, was uninterested in my research. They said, "We don't need this stuff. We're going to get this bill. It's all going to be wonderful." Surprise. It isn't all going to be wonderful. We *are* going to need all this information. We're going to have to do a class action suit in order to bomb the California Medical Board all to bits. Because they have absolutely no intention of letting midwives practice in a way that you and I would describe as authentic midwifery, whether you want to call it traditional or not.

One of the upsets about being prosecuted was that I had felt I was getting to a place in my life where I would be able to do the kinds of things that I wanted to do for myself, and then it was like being jerked back to ground zero, where I couldn't take the time to do anything I personally wanted to do. I could only raise money for legal defense and write letters to people.

I just don't believe that I could do what I do without having a very strong, well-developed religious vein. I really wonder about how other midwives handle these circumstances in which you just don't know how it's going to come out. I find myself praying for people, that whatever this mother needs will be there. Praying that guidance will come that will let me know when I need to do something different, like the mother with the ruptured membranes and thick meconium, that kind of stuff, that some wisdom that is higher than my conscious personality will allow me to see that there is a pattern here, and the direction it is leading me is the way to my goal. We constantly have to make choices about what is the right action to take, and how to make those choices I believe to be a religious activity. I'm saying, okay, God, give me some sense of it. You could have an almost equally compelling argument for intuition, except that there are instances which are beyond our intuition, which lie outside of ourselves as individual persons.

I think that God is creating us now, this instant. He's creating you and me and the consciousness that is going on between us right now. You're part of God, I'm part of God. It's all God. I believe that quality of being able to describe it internally as the loving father—and frankly, if anybody wants to consider God to be a loving mother, that's fine with me, too. But I personally find it very gratifying to feel like I'm the feminine, and God's the masculine. There's a verse from the Old Testament, a short one, that says, "My Maker is my husband." And that's the relationship I have with God. It's like He's there doing His part of the work, and I'm here doing my part of the work, and we're in this together. I would describe it that one is either codependent with one's fellow humans, or co-creative with God.

I think that a great deal of dysfunctional contemporary life is because I was expecting *you* to be God. If we don't have God anywhere else in our psyche, then we look to our relationships. You will protect me, you will keep me happy, whatever. We keep trying to pull God-ness out of the people around us, and in order to do that we manipulate, we enmesh, we enable, we do all these dysfunctional kinds of things. I think that the only other way to be in regard to the issue is to experience one's self as a co-creator. I believe that the aggregate statistic of the consciousness of the people who are alive this instant on the planet earth is what's going on here. If enough people hate their husband or their mother-in-law or the people next door to them, it manifests as great negativity. So I believe in that regard we are our brother's keeper, our mother's keeper, and our sister's keeper, and our children's keeper, and that we are not whole until we have acknowledged our connection with the Creator and with the created. That holiness is when we put ourselves in that place between God and our fellow human beings. I see myself as a servant, and I don't think that is a role that everybody has been assigned to, but I have been assigned to it.

I think that the language of it is pretty contemporary, but that the belief itself is part of my heritage. My particular religious heritage is one that should properly be called Judeo-Christian, I'm an Old Testament Christian. Another kind of subliminal background thing here is that I have always said, "Use me." I experience that I am somewhat unique in the context of midwifery in that I have had this long hospital experience. I don't have to wonder what would happen if we decided to dance with the devil. I've danced with the devil. I *know* what happens. And simultaneously I have a great deal of respect for Western medicine in regard to the kind of critical emergency circumstances under which it does so well. If you get hit by a truck, what you need is an ambulance, an IV [intravenous setup], and a real good ER [emergency room]/trauma center. I have seen babies born with a double cleft palate and sent them off with a pediatric surgeon and had them come back and look like normal babies. You want to send flowers because it's like a miracle. That's the part of medicine that I want to honor.

I've known individual people in medicine, doctors, obstetricians, that really are doing their best, and there's really this, for lack of a better word, a conspiracy against them, that a lot of obstetricians, particularly older ones, my age or older, who just gave up, kind of got drummed out of the corps. They spent their whole life thinking about this wonderful retirement party at the end of this great career, and instead they slink off in the middle of the

night because even the hospitals where they had privileges were harassing them because they were merely a doctor, they weren't an obstetrician.

One of the reasons why obstetricians have industrial-strength hate in regard to midwifery is that they spent a lot of time and energy running general practitioners out of maternity care. How could they run doctors out and then let nondoctors—midwives—practice? There's a real need to heal all these things. Healing and the concept of wholeness, bringing things back together. The answer is not bombing all the hospitals. It's how do we heal it? The obstetrician never sees a normal birth, is not trained in normal birth, does not experience normal birth—he can't imagine anybody doing homebirth—and he thinks that people who do homebirths are crazy. I understand that.

Physicians think that the way a woman gives birth is not so very important—"You've got the rest of your life." But midwives know that it matters when a woman herself gives birth, it matters that mothers hold and nurse their babies unhindered. Because if you fracture the parent/child bond, as doctors and nurses often do, you may well end up with a fractured parent and a fractured child. And it's the midwife's job to keep that fracture from happening, to keep them whole.

It is also the midwife's job to "midwife" the medical profession so that we can bring about a truly cooperative and complementary system of maternity care predicated on the practical well-being of mothers and babies. To accomplish that, midwives have to impersonally "love" a lot of doctors and be as patient and persistent with the medical profession as we are with our client families. I think that the story told about Eleanor Roosevelt, wife of President Roosevelt, describes this best. When Mrs. Roosevelt was asked by reporters who she put first, her children or her husband, she answered that "together with my husband, we put the children first." That characterizes the ideal relationship between midwives and physicians—that together we put the well-being of mothers and babies first.

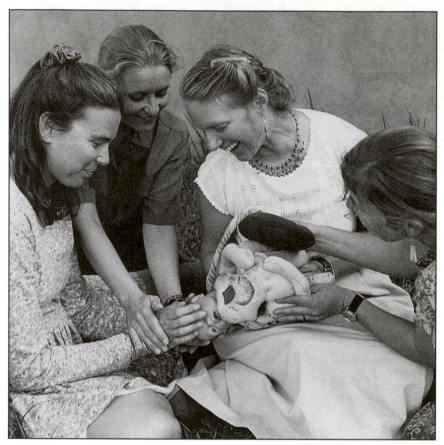

Elizabeth Gilmore

Elizabeth Gilmore is a licensed midwife in Taos, New Mexico, where she has a nationally accredited birth center called the Northern New Mexico Midwifery Center. Elizabeth has been training student midwives there since 1982 and has started a midwifery educational program called the National College of Midwifery. This is an at-a-distance learning program whereby midwives can complete educational modules at home and get their clinical experience with a local preceptor. The program also provides master's and Ph.D. levels of education. Elizabeth gave birth to three children at home, and only with the last did she have another midwife attend her. She attended her own daughter's birth in Thailand in 1992. Elizabeth is the founder and president of the Midwives Education Accreditation Council (MEAC), which was formed in 1991 to provide accreditation for midwifery programs in the United States. Elizabeth was involved in setting up licensing in New Mexico.

Elizabeth Gilmore

I started midwifery when I was twenty-three, so it's been about twenty-four years. I'm one of those people that didn't ever get any formal training. I was trained by mothers who were going to have their babies at home no matter what. These were really radical families that had done a lot of thinking about having control over their own births because those were the days when they were still using twilight sleep [a state in which awareness and memory of pain are dulled or blocked; produced by an injection of morphine and scopolamine]. I was a childbirth educator, and families would ask me to come take pictures. They would say, "You know more than we do." Presently I realized that people were treating me as if I knew more than I knew. So I told the doctors on Martha's Vineyard what I was doing, and they said, "This is really kind of awful, but since you're doing it, come to every birth at the hospital, and we'll show you everything we can, so you'll know when to bring people in." There were four of us who were childbirth educators. We were having our babies at about the same time, and we midwifed each other. People were birthing their own babies, but little by little people expected that I knew something, and at some point, I began to say, "You're doing great," and that's really what midwives do, as far as I'm concerned. I read everything I could, starting with *Williams Obstetrics* from my brother-in-law, who was a doctor.

Eventually I moved to New Mexico. I wasn't going to be a midwife, but when I came out here I got discovered and was asked if I could help

because they were going to make midwifery illegal. Another midwife recruited me to help write a pilot project to show that direct-entry midwifery in
New Mexico should be saved. In 1980 we had to get a public hearing to
create modern regulations. We started this birth center in 1982. This is the
only nationally accredited freestanding birth center run by direct-entry licensed, non–nurse-midwives. The study on birth centers that was done in
1989 included this and all kinds of birth centers, accredited and not [Rooks
et al. 1989]. The accreditation standards are hard to meet—there is much
paperwork, and it is very expensive.

Homebirths are safer, we have fewer transfers from home than from the
birth center. People are happier at home. The birth center is an intermediate
choice, for those who are not as confident in birth. We attend 60 percent of
our births here and 40 percent at home. The Hispanic moms come here
because they don't want blood in their homes. About 80 percent of our
moms are on Medicaid.

The native Americans receive free care and delivery if they go through
the Indian Health Service. They have to go to Santa Fe to birth in the hospital, so we only get two to four native American moms a year who are willing
to switch to Medicaid to come here. There are native American midwives,
older women and a very secret clan of women who deliver themselves. There
has been talk of having a birth center at the pueblo. I hope this happens.

A lot of people come to us for no good reason, just because "the midwives are pretty and they don't yell at us." We do PR [public relations] and
fundraising. We take care of people regardless of whether they can pay. We
have to raise between thirty thousand and sixty thousand dollars a year to
survive. An art auction brings the most money, because the artists here are
generous to a fault. And then we have the bake sales, small grants, and pledges.

It took me a while to learn not to bring my midwifery problems home. I
learned to not be so important, to let go, to present a midwifery service rather
than myself as the midwife. I learned to let students be the ones who did
intakes on the mothers so the moms would bond to the students; I learned to
take time off. That made all the difference, because then my family could
count on having me be free sometimes to be with them. I wouldn't have
survived as a midwife if I hadn't been able to make those changes. Older
midwives like myself have come to terms. They themselves are either constantly doing births, or they've switched to enabling other people to help at
birth. You choose one role or the other. Either you see yourself as the important person, or you let the mother or student take the lead.

Moms look up to us, and if we give an example of killing ourselves with work, then they'll do the same thing. I don't want to model that role. I love going to births still, after twenty-four years. When the phone rings at 3 A.M., I'm so happy.

Now my oldest daughter is twenty-four, and I delivered her daughter in Thailand two years ago in September. When the baby was in my hands I had this flood of feeling that I'd done everything now and I could die happy. I was by myself—I had understood that she would call her midwife, but she didn't. Just her husband was there, and he was so cute; "I'm first-time man to see baby born." He woke up the whole hotel. Everybody told me that I would be nervous because no one delivers family members—"You're going to goof." I'd been kind of flip until I got there, and began to feel really lonely. Then she was in labor saying, "Mom, this really hurts, I can't stand it anymore." "You're doing great," I replied, "you're about to deliver." And then I'd go into the bathroom and go, "Holy shit, I hope she's doing great!" She did fine.

I wanted to teach other midwives pretty much right away, because as a childbirth educator I was already teaching. Students, first of all, keep me learning all the time; their enthusiasm keeps me going. I find myself very isolated here in Taos. There aren't that many people like me, so students are peers. They are interested; they want to be midwives. By the time they make it to Taos to study to be midwives (which is hard to do because it's very expensive, it's out of the way, and it's not a big program), they're probably already midwives—they just need a place to manifest it.

To become a New Mexico licensed midwife takes a year and a half to two years if you're here and don't have access to more births. They study on their own, before they come or while they are here. We have classes on Wednesdays. Emergency skills are very important, but more than anything, I like to teach about confidence and trust and the ability to tell the difference between when things are fine and when they're not. It's important to know how to go through the steps to resolve stuff when it's not okay, to identify the clues, to use resources wisely.

Students don't have to become midwives for me. They're doing it for themselves. They come to me and tell me what they need, and I say, "Go right ahead." Ask me, do you want me to write your test? I get no bennies [benefits] out of how they're doing scholastically. I figure if they want to be midwives, they'll be midwives the best way they can, and if I can help I'm happy to. I'm pretty incidental. People have to be pretty motivated and self-

directed to study here. I make people come and spend three days with me so they can really see this is what it's going to be like. You have to jump right in, and you pretty much have to take care of yourself. It's not that I'm not here or don't care about you; I want you to participate. I'll help, but I'm not going to hand-feed you. You're doing this for yourself, not for me.

I feel so grateful that these students are willing to be midwives, to be with mothers when they are needed, that I'll often cry over things that are wonderful.

On Wednesdays we talk about what they want to know. We do chart review on Monday and agree on what needs to be done for each person. Depending on how experienced the students are, I'll have them do as much of seeing the people as they want to. I'm kind of an overwhelming person, and if I've done the visit, the moms just want to see me, so I try to stay in the background. I figure we're all students: the moms, the apprentices, and the midwives. The idea is that we all support each other. Most important are the moms. We teach the mother and her husband how to do BPs [blood pressure checks], urine tests, feel for position, listen to FHTs [fetal heart tones—the baby's heartbeat], as much as they want to do. We make a little chart that they can take home with them where they keep notes, so that they can really be involved. And then we have the family deliver the baby.

It is important for me to build community knowledge and to not have exclusive ownership of information. For example, saying, "Until you reach this level I cannot share my information with you," is something I think the medical educators and providers sometimes do. People who work in medicine tend to say, "I went to school for years, so until you do that I don't think we can talk." We need to let go of that authoritarian way of delivering care. You want to know about that, okay, here's the information. I think that would alleviate a great deal of the whole malpractice situation. Midwives are in a great place to start.

I love to study and to teach—I get a big kick out of it, seeing somebody light up with understanding. People ask me questions I haven't thought of. Why does the human body do this? What can we discover? Much of the time I'll have students teach the classes on Wednesday. I thought I might eventually work myself out of a job. If I teach the moms who come in here, they will just midwife each other. They'll call us for advice, but mothers and daughters and friends will eventually midwife each other.

At first the women that see me think that maybe I'm going to do it all to them. I say "Dipstick your urine, what does it say?" I take their word for

it—I don't double-check them either. I want them to get the idea that "you're the one who's going to be doing this." I really want them to have confidence.

My interest in organizational stuff came from being chair of the education committee for the New Mexico Midwives Association (NMMA). They asked me as the chair to please resolve two problems with midwifery education in New Mexico. One was there was no status, no degree, and two was there was no uniform curriculum. I came up with the idea of a college, the National College of Midwifery. Because I'm interested in education, I was going to the National Coalition of Midwifery Education meetings, and they were the ones who suggested that I make this a national program. They said, "We all want access to this kind of ability to get a degree. All you have to do is change a little bit of the entry requirements." NMMA voted to go ahead, and New Mexico would take care of the administration. It came about rather innocently; we've gotten a good response and are seeking national accreditation.

It is a very hard program to do, because it's very comprehensive and you do it all yourself with a preceptor. But we've had our first graduates for associate's degrees and B.S. degrees. As part of the program you need to conduct research in the field. We want to know from midwives: What are you doing? Is it working and why? When it's in research format people who aren't midwives can also understand it.

Midwives' personalities are so overwhelming—it's been astonishing to me. The very first time I noticed it was when I was a childbirth educator, and I had very strong ideas about how a person should birth. I have realized since that I do midwifery for myself, and I should do it actively for myself instead of unconsciously. That's one of the biggest things I teach students, too. I never want to hear, "After all I've done for her, she was ungrateful."

Every day when you go in to be a midwife it's because you enjoy it, you're mostly benefiting yourself; education lets you channel your endeavors so that the woman benefits too. Life is very short and unpredictable. Saying you're doing something only for somebody else is being stuck up and inaccurate. Moms don't owe you a thing—except money! I love hugs and kisses, if they come from people being happy because *they* succeeded, not because I was magic.

I'm a rare person in that I can remember my own birth. I had a great birth experience. I can even see the doctor, the room. With *my* first baby I was in labor for thirty-two hours. There was nobody to help me at home but

my husband, my sister, my books, and a neighbor who had visited the Frontier School of Nursing in the 1940s. We went to the hospital and I delivered in half an hour. The doctor was going to give me drugs and I said, "I'll just get up and leave." The nurse left. He said, "Your husband and sister have to leave." "Fine," I said, "I'm leaving with them." When the baby was born, I said, "Give her to me." Well, he was flabbergasted that my daughter would nurse, because he'd never seen a birth without scopolamine or Demerol. He got to see it happen. He asked me to teach other ladies.

My second birth I had at home, and it was very easy, a day long but not hard. I wanted to just stay in the dark and have the baby, but I felt compelled to come down and birth with the family. For my third baby my mother invited me to come down to Mexico and have it at her house and she would take care of me. It sounded like a glorious vacation, so I took my midwife with me. My midwife, my ex-husband, my new husband, and my two children went down in our camper. My midwife had been kind of sick, so I didn't call her until three or four minutes before the birth. This was the first birth where I wasn't responsible, so when the baby was a little floppy [needed resuscitating] I just handed him to her and said, "Here, you do that." It was great to not have to take care of everyone else while I was taking care of myself. At my other births I had to be really vigilant because I was the only one who knew what was going on, but with this one I could relax.

I pray at difficult births—"Dear God, please look down on this lovely woman and let it be all right. Please help us." I pray inside, in a very childish way, like when I was five or six. I revert to this childish wish that the universe will protect this woman and the ones I love. And sometimes I will kneel down and kiss the ground when something great happens and say, "Thank you, this is totally cool. I'm really grateful."

There are times I try to do magic, like when I take off my necklace because somebody isn't dilating, and put it on the bed and open it. Just to make me feel better. Not with any real expectations it will work.

I've had my hair stand up on end, I've been so scared at some births. I'm sort of like a bulldog, and when I have to act, I will, and I'm mean and harsh and really get in there and do something that has to be done. It's great to be able to be laid back and not do anything if you don't have to, but it's also great to be able to do things that have to be done. Like remove a placenta manually, or start an IV [intravenous line], intubate [insertion of a tube into the respiratory tract to create a clear airway] a baby, suck out all that meconium [the baby's first stool; it is sticky and dangerous for the baby to

inhale at birth] and resuscitate them. I'll get in a special mindset—I will do it, no doubt. The doubt is right before I begin.

Some students can't do that right away. Then you teach them. "This is how I usually do it—I make up my mind, I know I'm going to be able to do this." You hand them the stuff and say, "Here *you* do this." It's a crisis for them. It brings out the adrenaline. I think it's great practice to start IVs and take blood. If they can do that they can do anything. If they can overcome their fear of not getting the vein, nothing else is as hard as that first time.

I'm just a nut for midwifery, and I'm so grateful for anybody else who is a midwife. I'm one of these people that can attend a birth and I forget it. You could ask me about the birth I did three days ago, and I could maybe not remember many details about it without looking at the chart. I'm there and then I'm gone, moving on to the next thing. I very often don't remember who did the birth. I was just *there*.

One of the things that has fascinated me over the years is that I recognize the children's faces. I've noticed that I can look at a fifteen-year-old and I can say, "I delivered you!" and I've been so surprised to recognize them, especially as I don't get very attached to the babies, I'm mostly attached to their mothers.

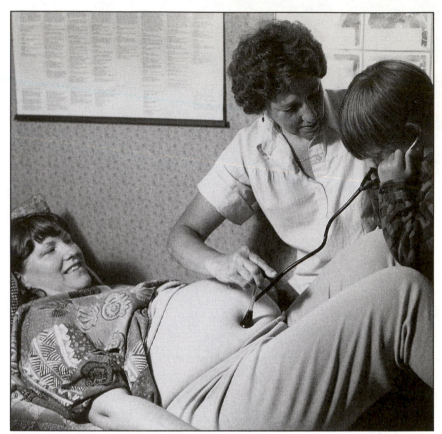

Tina Guy

Tina Guy is a nurse-midwife who lives in Dresden, Maine. She received her midwifery training at the Frontier School of Midwifery and Family Nursing in 1976. She is presently in a graduate program in nursing at the University of Southern Maine and working on a project with pregnant and parenting teens. She worked at a birth center in Wiscasset, Maine, from 1981 to 1991, until the birth center closed due to lack of support from the medical community. She attended homebirths, sometimes with a lay midwife, for a number of years. Because there were no midwives working in hospitals in her area (and there are other good midwives in her area who still attend homebirths) she has joined an obstetrician to attend births in a hospital in Brunswick, Maine. She also has worked at the Kennebec Women's Health Center for the past fourteen years. Tina is active in the Maine Chapter of ACNM, the Maine State Nurses Association, Sigma Theta Tau (the nursing honor society), and the Midwives of Maine. She is teaching in a lay midwifery program called Birthwise.

Tina Guy

My son Alex was born in our front bedroom, in the bed that belonged to my husband's great-grandparents. Bob's mom was born in that bed, and we decided it had good vibes. Actually Alex is adopted. His birth mom is a friend of my good friend. Bob and I weren't going to have kids, but my friend told me about this woman who was due in two months who wanted a private adoption because she wanted some say in who her son would be with. We had talked about adopting a child and then we decided not to, and I thought maybe this was just meant to be. We were renovating our house upstairs—it was as if we knew we were going to have a baby and had to have an upstairs that was warmer. So Bob was working on tearing out the walls while I talked to the birth mother on the phone for over an hour that first time. We'd never even met each other before. We were talking about the things that we liked and where we were coming from. We talked a little about why she was giving the baby up for adoption and who the baby's father was, and if he was healthy and if she was healthy, and had she had any prenatal care during this pregnancy. We just talked about all kinds of things. We decided we would go down and meet her. When we met her and her other two kids, we just immediately clicked. She looks like my little sister, with dark hair. When Alex was born, he looked like baby pictures of me.

After Alex was born I nursed him. I had been pumping my breasts for two months using a battery-run breast pump, and he never lost any weight. For about the first four months he would come with me to births—he was

very good. Even if he was fussy or cranky, right at the time the birth was getting serious, when the woman was really pushing the baby out, he would calm down and watch and watch and watch. And as soon as the baby was born and cried, he fell asleep. It was as if all the tension were gone.

So that went on for about four months until he was older and more intrusive to the woman's space. So I left him at home when I had to be gone for two nights at a birth. When I came home he refused to nurse. I was in tears, but we gave it up. I was really lucky that when I decided to leave him, we had a second assistant at the birth center who became his babysitter. So on the way to the birthing center I'd drop him off, and after the birth, we'd call her and she'd bring Alex over to the birthing center and she would do the cleaning up and all that stuff. There is an older woman in her seventies who takes care of him now. Bob can call her at 6 A.M. and say, "Tina has gone to a birth, can you take care of Alex?" and she says, "Sure, no problem." She lives just a mile away.

I met my husband at a big summer cookout. Somehow, there were these two men talking about homebirth, and as I walked by one grabbed me and said, "Here she is, this is my midwife." And Bob looked at me, he's an archaeologist, and said, "Midwife? I didn't know they existed anymore. That's fascinating, we have to talk." We met in July and knew in the first week of November we were going to get married, and I said, "Are you sure you want to do this? You know the life of a midwife is crazy." And he said, "Tina, nothing could have been crazier than this September. . . ." I had eleven homebirths the September before we got married.

One of the first births I ever saw was a nurse-midwife delivery, with a West Indian midwife. There was an instructor and five students standing at the end of this delivery table and we had gotten the woman's permission to be there. It was wonderful; I just remembered having tears in my eyes. The whole bunch of us were all choked up—even the instructor—and I remember she said, "Don't be embarrassed, I do this every time I see a birth." She loved obstetrics so much it carried over to us. Birth wasn't as awful as I thought it was going to be. Then I saw a couple of physician's deliveries and I was really sure that midwives delivered babies better, or in a more humane way. I saw a battle between a midwife and a resident at a hospital: this poor woman was in labor, and the midwife felt that something either needed to be done or not to be done, and the resident disagreed with her. And the upshot was, she said, "This woman is my client, get out of the delivery room," and I thought, Wow, what a powerful woman, and he left. I thought, I wonder if

midwifery makes women this way or if it's women who are that way go into midwifery, so I just started checking things out more.

I think that being a midwife has definitely made me more of a feminist, and more of a powerful woman. I really come across as being powerful, and some people decide not to use me as a midwife because they are afraid I'll use my power to be too controlling. But I try really hard in my midwifery practice not to do that, especially at births, because it is such an important time that women need to develop their own power. And if they have a good birth experience, whether they end up with a C-section or forceps or a vaginal birth without any interference, it makes them a more powerful, centered, complete person, so that's what I try to do as a midwife. And I do step in and make my opinions known when they need to be, but other than that, I try to support what the woman needs to do. For instance, delivering in whatever crazy position she needs to, as long as the baby is not going to fall on the floor. And the first time I ever assisted a woman who delivered on hands and knees, I thought, "I don't know which way is up!"

I tend to be semiradical as a nurse-midwife. I have worked with a lay midwife who had a phenomenal belief in a woman's ability to give birth. She's very spiritual—there was something that was really different. We'd be in situations where we would be at a birth at home, and I'd look at her and say, "I don't know—what do you think?" and she'd say "She'll do it." It always seemed to be when I wasn't confident she would be, and when she wasn't confident I would be, and when we both were not confident, we would go into the hospital. I think that it's really helpful in being a midwife to be able to listen to your intuition, to listen to your gut. I think that for the most part it makes you be a more successful midwife. When I'm really fearful, I act on my fear. And if my fear doesn't go away when I think it should, and even though there isn't anything you can measure or pinpoint, and my stomach starts doing weird things, then as far as I'm concerned it's time to not be at home and to transfer to the hospital. The first time that ever happened to me, I was doing homebirths and I was with a woman who was in labor for a little over a day. She was making progress and we checked her again, her blood pressure was okay and all of a sudden I felt as if there was this black cloud of doom that was hanging over my head, and I was really nervous. I just felt we needed to get out of here. So I called my backup doc and said, "I don't know what it is, Jim. She looks okay right now. She's dilating really slowly. I just don't want to be home with her anymore, I want to come in."

And he said fine and we went in, and two hours after we got to the

hospital, her blood pressure skyrocketed. She looked up at us and said, "I feel really strange." She didn't have a convulsion because we jumped on it so fast, but I think she was headed for severe toxemia [a pregnancy-related condition associated with high blood pressure, swelling, and protein in the urine; it can lead to serious complications including maternal convulsions]. There was no indication at home. So after that I thought, yep, listen to your instincts, Tina. Because when Jim said, "You are a lucky kiddo. Why did you bring her in here?" And I said, "I don't know. My gut said she needed to be here."

I really think that the medical establishment has done a great disservice to women in the whole area of birth. I think it's great all the advances we have for high-risk pregnancies and for high-risk babies. It's fantastic how we can save moms and save babies. And if you have a labor that is dragging on you can use pitocin and get that baby out before a problem. But what I've seen happening in the medical community is this increased use of technology when it's not warranted—almost talking women into complications. I get really angry about it. The insurance companies are also getting involved now and telling the doctors and midwives what to do and what they don't have to do. And if you don't practice the way they say you should practice then they take your insurance from you. I have some real problems with the use of technology and forcing people to practice the way that they really don't believe. I have to practice in a more defensive way as a homebirth nurse-midwife now to keep my backup, I can't be that laid back anymore.

I have a set of protocols that says if I have someone with ruptured membranes for over twenty-four hours that have been documented then they have to be in the hospital. And I disagree with that because I have seen so many times that after three or four or five days with no internal exams, they go into labor and have a fine labor. The baby is fine and the mom is fine.

When you are an insecure midwife you have a lot more transfers, because you are transferring before you really need to, or you are transferring because the clients are picking up on your insecurity and they become insecure and scared. It can slow down their labors. Or because you are expecting complications, they occur. When I was working at the birthing center from eighty-two to eighty-six, we had two C-secs and five transfers out of a total of 150 births. It was just phenomenal. When another midwife started working with me and we began experiencing lots of negativity from the local medical establishment, our C-section rate went to about 20 percent. Part of this was her insecurity, and part of it was mine too, all the nasty stuff that was going on, with everyone on our case because they felt we weren't transferring soon

enough even though we were still practicing under the same protocols we had used since 1982. So we ended up with a lot more complications and a lot more C-sections. I think our clients picked up on our paranoia about the local medical system. The birth center was also being badmouthed for our decisions—it didn't matter what kind of decision we made. No matter what we did it was wrong—it was a climate that was just waiting for something to happen.

After seven years of trying to convince the doctors that we were practicing safely and doing a fairly good job, a new obstetrician moved in and the situation deteriorated. She was determined to find something wrong with how we practiced even if she had to mostly manufacture it. And I just got tired of fighting, and we had to close the birth center.

My theory about birth in this country is that we've bred passivity into women as far as how they participate in the birth experience. It is almost as if women don't do what they really need to because they've heard so many bad birth stories and that you are supposed to stay in bed. Or they've had a hospital birth experience that when their water has broken and they are supposed to stay in bed, they weren't allowed to even get out of bed to go to the bathroom even if the baby's head was down low. It is as if they need to be given permission to do some of these things.

The hardest part of being a midwife is lack of sleep. The crazy hours and having to drive in all kinds of rotten, stressful weather to births has affected my health. For a while I had sciatica that was almost crippling. It is amazing, I think that midwives take care of other people so much that they neglect themselves sometimes. So I decided about a year ago that I would stop neglecting myself and take care of myself, so I've started going to a chiropractor and a massage therapist, and it's really made a huge difference. This year the sciatica is still there but I'm so much better. Here I am trying to do all these things, and if I'm feeling like this now what is it going to be like when I'm sixty—or seventy or eighty—if I'm still around?

I could do a lot more births, but I'm going to school. My grandmother said to me one time, "Tina, you will always be in school, you are a perennial student." I was one of the first people in my family to ever go to college. I came from a typical blue-collar family, Irish Catholic, where all the girls got married and had lots of kids except for me.

Full-time school went down the drain due to finances, so what I'm doing is going part-time for a master's in nursing. I want to teach, and ideally what I want to see is a midwifery school get started in Maine. The medical

community feels that you really need the credentials, and if you're not accepted by the medical community the students are not going to get the experience that they need. There are only so many people doing homebirths, so you've got to be able to work with physicians who are willing to have students come in to the hospital too.

I'm very positive about things, that's why I love homebirths, and why I feel I exude confidence about homebirths. There are some people who say, How can you deliver people at home, what if something happens . . . ? If something happens, it happens and we deal with it then. I have seen what happens in the hospital, and I know that at the birthing center and at home I watch people a lot more closely than they do in many hospitals. I take blood pressures more often. I listen to the baby's heart rate more often. I'm always panicking in the hospital and asking the nurse to get the heart rate for me because it is not being done often enough. I guess people get cocky in the hospital and say, "Oh, we're here . . ."

As midwives we feel as if we need to be everything to everybody, and over the years I've realized I can't be everything to everybody. And I'm not always going to be perfect and everything I do may not be right—that's something that doctors need to learn. Because they jump all over midwives for things that midwives are doing—when they do some absolutely outrageous things themselves.

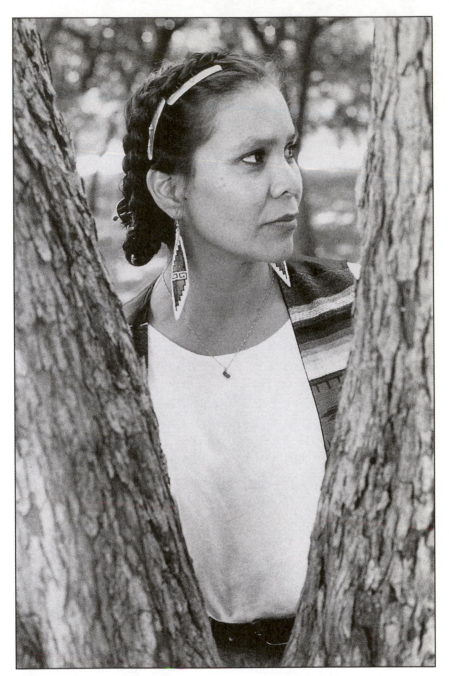

Toni House

Toni House is from the Oneida Nation in Wisconsin and is the mother of two young children. She serves as a facilitator and trainer in all of the different tribal programs. She has a master's in counseling and has worked as a psychotherapist for the Oneida Tribe for five years prior to her current position. She follows in the footsteps of her great-grandmother in her work as a midwife.

Toni House

What inspired me to learn midwifery was hearing Jeannie Shenandoah, a midwife from the Iroquois Nation, talk at a Year of the Child conference back in seventy-eight in Washington State. She spoke about women learning to take care of their bodies and being self-sufficient. And that as Indian people we are sovereign nations, and that being self-sufficient included birthing our own children in the natural childbirth setting. I believe I was sixteen, and I'd always been in that movement of learning who I am and knowing my ways. At that point I had been preparing myself all through high school to be a nurse, and when I heard Jeannie I thought, That's right down my alley, back to what the Creator wants us to be like. I wouldn't be going into the education system, to be like a nurse, and supporting that kind of economy and social lifestyle, but I would be promoting self-sufficiency and knowing who we are as aboriginal people and knowing about our bodies, knowing the best foods—it's like an overall balance. So that's when I decided I wanted to be a midwife.

There are two connections from my childhood to midwifery that I can think of. My mother told me this after I became a midwife: "Back in the late fifties and sixties, when I was having you, everyone got these shots and got put to sleep while they delivered your baby. When you were born, I don't know why, I insisted on having a natural birth. They weren't promoting that at that time."

She was out in California by herself, didn't know anything about having

children, or about her body. She just kept having these babies as she always described it to me. She had four children at that time with my father. One baby every year.

"And for some reason, I just would not let them give me medication. You must have known then. You must have given me some message that you were going to be born that way."

Growing up, my mother always talked to me about taking care of my body. My mother was young and came from a very poor family, got married very young, one of her parents died when she was a little girl, it was real hard on her. I'd always ask her questions about her body. I was the only girl of four, and I was the youngest, so I'd always be in the bathroom with her, talking and talking. If I saw her stretchmarks, I'd ask, and she'd say, "That's from having babies and not knowing how to take care of myself. When you grow up you're going to know that you don't have to have babies if you don't want to. You're going to know how to take care of yourself, how to eat, all those things. You're not going to end up like me."

Then she had my little sister when I was twelve. She'd had one of those shaves, a prep, and I'm twelve years old and still in the bathroom, "Ma, what happened, how come you look like that?" She says, "When you have a baby, they shave you." I thought it was so ugly. Then she gives me that thing, "When you get older, you're going to know." She always told me that. She had a lot of faith in me. She put a lot of her dreams in me. "I really believe," she always said, "you're going to be this, be that. You're Indian, and you'll always remember who you are. Indian first, before anything. Learn our ways, about self-sufficiency." I think she just ingrained me. And then when I said I wanted to be a nurse, she thought that was really nice. The day I said I wanted to be a midwife, she said, "Oh, I'm going to tell Jeannie."

My mother was good friends with Jeannie, and when Jeannie came to visit us she gave me Margaret Nofziger's book on contraception [*A Cooperative Method of Natural Birth Control*], and *Our Bodies, Ourselves*. Jeannie said, "Start reading. That's what you're going to have to do, is read, read, read." I didn't hear from her until I was nineteen. She called me up and she said, "You still want to be a midwife? We want to send someone to Tennessee, to The Farm." "Yes!" I said. I went.

The following year after that, she said, "You know, you're single, you don't have children, you don't have a family. You'd be the best person to go off and continue your midwifery training. Then you can bring it back to your community. We would like to send you to El Paso." She had a grant through

a foundation (Seven Generation Fund) and they funded me to go to El Paso. That's how I got started, when I was twenty-one.

I was in college at the time. I thought, I'm going to get me a good basis for midwifery, so I was taking the sciences and nutrition and anything on human development. When they told me they would fund me to El Paso, I wrote up my independent study under the midwifery and the human development area. So I got twenty-seven credits for midwifery studies as independent study. I used all my schoolwork from El Paso, and each semester I got twelve more, and afterward I went to the Yucatan and wrote a paper on the social history of the Yucatan and then did another independent study on Hispanic *curanderas* [traditional healers] of Mexico. When I came back I wrote an independent study on Hispanic midwives, so all together I got thirty credits undergraduate from midwifery. I designed my own degree in human development with a special emphasis on midwifery.

My own birth experiences and children have taught me so much—it almost should be a prerequisite to midwifery, although the discipline and time you have to devote to midwifery is difficult once you have a family. I had learned a sensitivity from being with women several years before I had children, but all of a sudden when you get pregnant, you get all these questions. You want to know everything, and I learned a lot through my own childbirth experience.

The biggest lesson I learned was the power of spirit—what I always equated with the power of God. As midwives we see that at every delivery. There are these little spirits that are always around you. Different people see them different ways, but in birth, in transition, it's just like when God enters you. You shake because the power is so enormous. You get nauseated, get sick because the power is so strong. You lose all control of everything. That's usually when the woman says, "I can't do it." Then you know the baby is going to come, as soon as a woman lets go of her control, God comes in, the power and the spirit comes in birth. That's how I see it.

So when I was able to do that with my children—with the second one I did much better—I felt the power of God. I felt like a spiritual shift happening. I think as midwives we're honored with that opportunity to be present when that happens. I guess that's basically what I've learned. I always recognized it, but I didn't understand it as much until now.

I guess the second thing that I learned is the power of women. Dealing with people and emotions, with the spirit you learn intuition. I learned intuition from midwifery. Any animal has that, and we're animals. It brings you

back to your natural origins and instincts. But our society doesn't promote that. In kindergarten we don't encourage our children to stay in touch with their natural instincts and intuitions. You relearn it later, maybe as a mother, but through midwifery you learn intuition and the power of it.

For me to become a midwife was a desire, but the opportunity came easy. I thought if it came that easy, then the Creator must have put it there. It must be meant to be, so I picked it up, and every time I picked it up, something else would come, so I picked that up. I always believed that if you're going down the path the Creator has given to us, certain "right" things will present themselves. You have to be determined and have your eyes open so you can see it, but it'll come to you. And everything has always just presented itself. I never had to look too hard for different things. Of course, I had to work hard once I got there, but if I wanted to go to a conference or something, it came. If I wanted to go to school, it came. I always figured the Creator laid that down for me and watched to see if I figured it out. I could have gone and not picked it out, but I don't think my life would have been the way it was planned. The way I've been taught through my people's teachings is that we already know what we're coming here to do before we get here. I think the Creator has given me real good eyes to see, so that's what I do.

I never, ever wanted to be a psychotherapist. All of a sudden it's knocking on my door, and I'm like, no. Then everything starts coming, and it's just like they came and got me. I tried to resist it for some time, and people kept knocking on my door. I had no interest in being a counselor.

So when I was working with kids, social services recruited me for the tribe, and the University of Wisconsin—Oshkosh gave me a scholarship to go for my master's in counseling. When I got there, my main teacher was one of those magical people. He told me counseling is an art and some people are gifted with it. "Your art is counseling."

I said, "No way. I'm just doing this to help my midwifing. This will help me work with families because I always deal with emotional problems in some way or another when attending a woman in childbirth. I always get this emotional stuff when I thought I was just there to help get the baby out."

And he said, "Well, I don't know what you're meant to do with it, but you're meant to do it. You got something there." So I did counseling for five years and kept praying to God that this wasn't going to be my life. But what I think made counseling natural for me was the second gift that I learned from midwifery. When you deal with midwifery, you learn about your gut, and you

learn to trust your instincts. So that in counseling if you trust your gut and your instincts, you can go anywhere you want with people—wherever they want to let you go. They'll only go as much as they're ready. It's just like in birth. They'll only go when they're ready, whenever that time is right. Not when I want it, when they want, but whenever the time is right. That's how counseling is.

So a lot of times I compare birth and counseling. Just like when you get to transition; I'd always say to my women, you know how scary it is, and you feel like you can't go on, and you just give up, and then it comes, the baby comes, and you're beautiful, and everyone talks about how scary it is. Life is just like that in every single moment. It's birth, all the time. The only difference is that birth is just more apparent, and death, of course.

I don't know, I think that all midwives have the potential to be that fluid to be a counselor or a midwife. If you are a very good midwife and if you can trust that intuitiveness, you can do it. That's all it is, working with people, it's just trusting your instinct, your gut. This is just my theory. I don't really know, because I'm still young in my path. I'm not doing as much birthing as I was, and I think somehow I needed that counseling part to balance that, and that I'm going to get a calling to go back to midwifery. I don't think it's right now. I think the Creator is having me do all these different things and I don't know how they come together, but I trust that what I'm going to evolve into is going to be something old.

The biggest challenge for me in midwifery was having people take me seriously, and being so young. I'd walk in and they'd kind of laugh. Oh, ain't she cute. In a lot of ways definitely it's true that only the old women used to have midwifery skills. In our ways, there were the older women, and it was their wisdom that helped laboring women, and I was young, and I didn't have wisdom yet. I had something, but not what an older woman would have. They always said, you'll never be a midwife. And at some point, even after I came out of El Paso's Maternity Center, I believed them. It took me two years to realize I already was, and there was no stopping it.

Right now if people insist on having me, I wouldn't turn them away, but if I can persuade them to go somewhere else, to another midwife, I will. I'll sway them that way, but if they insist on having me, there's no way I'd turn them away. That's the way I feel. When you have a gift I don't think that it is my right to say no, because I think the Creator gave it to me, and that's the way it is. Sometimes I think, well, maybe I'm just not going to be doing midwifery anymore, because He hasn't called. And I'll get a call the next day

and they'll say, "We don't want no one else. We just want you." "Are you sure? Okay."

So I think the Creator gives me little breaks, but just always reminding me in some way in my life all the time, I'm just taking a little break, and I still have to do this. I don't think I'll ever not do midwifery completely. I'm not going to say I'm done with this. That's not ever going to happen until I die. You always do it in some sense.

But I hope it will be a while before I feel that call again, because it's such a heavy responsibility. I'd like to be with my own family for a while, maturing my self, and become that old wise woman some day, and then dedicate my life to midwifery if that's what's meant in the cards. The one thing that I'm pretty sure I know in my heart, I can't ever not do it.

When things are going good I try to always remember to pray, because when things are going bad you want Him to hear you then, too. Fear at births helps give me my connection to the Creator. It's like telling God you have no control over that. You can only do the best you can, and the power of prayer takes you. Sometimes you don't know what you're doing, but you go through that dark curtain, dark cloud, and that's why you don't want to go, because you don't know what's on the other side. You go through that door, and all you have is a prayer. That's how birth is. All you have is a prayer. You can always be learning and studying and have all these experiences with other midwives and teachers, but when it's right down there you can only do the best you can, and that's all you got, and everything else you're not in control of it. You're like a facilitator, and you can do the best you can with all the resources you know, your brain and your intuitiveness, but we don't have control of the rest, so that's when the power of prayer is the best thing you've got.

I don't know why, but when I was in really hard births, I thought of my ancestors, my grandmothers. I don't know if it was because it was them who came and helped me out when I needed that little bit of assistance. I don't know if they are there with me, but that's who I think of. My grandmother pretty much raised me, and her grandmother was a midwife—my great-great-grandmother. I didn't know she was a midwife until the year I went to school. My grandmother told me a story that her grandmother, who knew a lot about herbs, had said to her, "Now you remember these things that I tell you, because some day someone's going to ask you, and you're going to need to remember." My gramma told me this two years ago when I said, "Gramma, remember! Can't you remember that?"

She just shook, and she said, "I can't believe this is happening."
"What?" "My grandmother, she used to tell me," and she told me in Indian
what the word was, "she used to shake her finger and say in Indian, 'now you
remember.' Never did I ever think it would be my own granddaughter." That
was real special. When I think of birth, I think of my grandmothers. I always
do, and I just pray and give them acknowledgment.

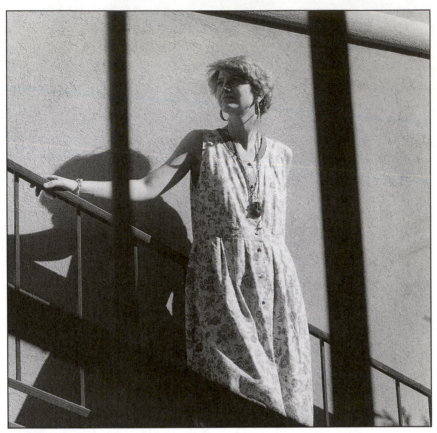

Kaye Kanne

Kaye Kanne received her midwifery training from the Birthways Midwifery School in La Mesa, New Mexico, and the Maternity Center in El Paso, Texas. After being licensed in New Mexico and trained as an emergency medical technician (EMT), she then moved to Alaska, where she set up a homebirth practice. In 1985 she started work to pass legislation that would recognize midwifery as a legal profession. This was to counter attempts by the Alaska Medical Association to get a court ruling that delivering babies is included in the practice of medicine. Midwives had been regulated by the Department of Health and Social Services, whose regulations were so restrictive as to eliminate midwifery practice in Alaska. After seven years of the midwives' and their supportive clients' hard work, in 1992 the Midwives Association of Alaska was successful in creating a separate board of midwifery for certified direct-entry midwives to practice in homes and to independently run birth centers. Kaye lives in Juneau with her husband and five children. She has been chair of the Alaska state licensing board since it was created in 1992.

Kaye Kanne

I got into midwifery after having my own babies. I had my first baby when I was twenty and I was very naive. I knew absolutely nothing. I didn't take any classes. I didn't read any books except for skimming a Lamaze book. I thought, "Everybody has babies. They come out." My doctor would just pat me on the head and say, "Don't worry about a thing," if I asked any questions. I really wasn't concerned about it at all. I was pretty healthy in spite of the fact that my diet was typically American. I went into the hospital and had a typical American birth at that time, in 1976. I had a spinal and was numb from the waist down. I had Demerol before that. I was totally alone during my labor. I had no support. My husband wasn't allowed in. I was flat on my back, with my legs in the stirrups, and had a huge episiotomy. The spinal was given to me four minutes before my baby was born. It took four hours to wear off, and then I got a spinal headache [a side effect of anesthesia]. I didn't see my baby during that time because I reacted to the spinal. I was very scared. I just thought that I felt bad, because I had done something wrong. It was my fault that I was having such a bad time, because I wasn't prepared. I wanted to breastfeed my baby and it was really hard for me. I didn't have any support for that. It took me about four days to figure it out. They finally said, "You can't go home unless this baby latches on" [on to the breast for breast-feeding], but they had been giving him bottles in the nursery. Finally he latched on, and we went home. It was just really, really hard. I never felt

complete with that experience. I didn't feel good about it, but I felt like it was my fault, like I hadn't done something right.

The next time that I got pregnant, two-and-a-half years later, I decided that I wanted to do natural childbirth. It was really scary for me to think about doing it that way since it had been so hard with all the drugs. What would a natural childbirth be like? So I started reading books—I must have read twenty of them. I guess all the right books just fell into my hands, like Suzanne Arms's *Immaculate Deception.*

I evolved from wanting to have a natural childbirth to wanting to have a homebirth. It took me at least half of the pregnancy to figure out what a midwife was. I didn't know they existed. I called a lot of doctors, asking if they would do a homebirth. Finally, one told me to call a midwife. I said, "What's a midwife?" I found a wonderful midwife who would come to my home and do prenatal care. She taught me how to eat. I didn't know anything about nutrition before that. During that pregnancy, I changed my life one hundred and eighty degrees. I started changing and growing. It was definitely a transformation. I attended three different childbirth classes. My husband wasn't very supportive. His attitude was that if you really want to do this, I guess I'll be there.

I had a wonderful experience. My mom was there, and I had a great midwife. Labor is never easy, but it was a wonderful and empowering labor. I think that whole experience changed my life. I'm much stronger than I ever would have been. That's why I do what I do, because of that empowerment of women when they have that kind of experience, taking that kind of responsibility. Later I had a little girl whose birth at home was very, very difficult because she was almost ten pounds. Again, that was very empowering. That was six years later, with a different husband and I was living in Juneau, Alaska, and was practicing midwifery by then.

I think that bonding is very important. That first four hours that I wasn't with my first son has made a tremendous difference in our relationship. Bonding is just crucial. The first few minutes, the first hour, I'm not saying that you can't be a good parent, because I feel like I've been a good parent, but it's been difficult. You have to parent more from an intellectual, emotional place, rather than an instinctual place. If you're bonded with that baby from the time of birth on, if you're not separated, it's more of an instinct. It's more of just a knowing. It's much, much different, the relationship. I see that, not just in relationship to my own children, but in other

women who have been through the same thing. I believe that we bond with our babies after birth on an emotional, spiritual, and physical level. The emotional and spiritual can be made up for later, but the physical is just not there. Breastfeeding helps. I think it makes a difference in their self-image, how they see themselves in the world. My first child was very fearful, and independent at a very early age. He learned very early on that his needs were not going to be met because of the way I was parenting him. *Better Homes and Gardens* says that if your baby doesn't need to be changed or nursed or whatever, you shouldn't hold them all the time. I really tried to do what the book said. I was very young. I didn't know. I didn't have the support system. I would pick him up when he was crying and I would feel very guilty. It was really difficult. I breastfed for only six months, because I didn't have the support from many women around me.

With my second child I nursed him for the first twenty-four hours, nonstop. He was very dependent for a year, then he was very independent. He was very sure of himself. It's some kind of inner sense of strength that kids who aren't bonded with their parents just don't have. My daughter, I nursed her until she was three. She was very dependent until she was two and a half. She would nurse even during the night several times, but she is so strong, so sure of herself in this world. I can see the difference. It's amazing. She won't have to do as much counseling when she's older.

As soon as my second child was born I started thinking about becoming a midwife, yet felt that I could never do that—being in total awe of midwives. I was living in Portland, Oregon, and became a childbirth educator and got very political with a natural birth association. For three-and-a-half years I did everything I could to attend births—I would take pictures, do child care, or labor coach—whatever. I studied and went to every workshop they had at the time.

I did feel that midwifery was hard to get into and that midwives were very cliquish. We moved to New Mexico for me to get my midwifery training, and then we moved to Juneau, Alaska. When I got there I basically set up my own practice and joined a midwife who had been attending births for about ten years. She came from the background of being an EMT and having a degree in women's studies. Friends had asked her to be at their births, and she evolved into being the local midwife.

I do between twenty and thirty births a year—between two and four births a month. I work with an upper-middle-class population mostly—a lot of state government workers, attorneys—and with many from the fishing community. The native people in Juneau have a clinic where their health care is paid

for 100 percent. I have worked with a few native women who have wanted to have homebirths, but most of them birth in the hospital where it is paid for.

The hardest thing about living here is that it rains so much—over one hundred inches a year. We don't see the sun a lot and people get depressed. Also, being so isolated and far away from other midwives is hard. The rest of Alaska is just as far away as Seattle. You can get to Juneau only by boat or by plane, so it's hard to go anywhere financially. I can't even go to a midwifery conference in Anchorage when I have people due because it's too far.

I lobbied very hard for midwifery legislation in 1985. I thought that it was very important to have consistent standards for care for midwives practicing in this state. I think that in order to be recognized as professionals, instead of "I catch babies," that we need regulations and we need licensure. I've gone round and round about it, because in Alaska, we did get a bill passed in 1985 for regulation in the Department of Health and Social Services, and then six years later we still don't have regulations in place. Health and Social Services has had an attitude; one, we don't want the liability, we don't want to do this, if we're pressured into putting these regulations in place, then we're going to make regulations that make it impossible for people to practice, because we don't want to do this. Another prevalent attitude is that it is our job to protect the public from midwives. That's how they see regulation. I don't see regulation like that. I see regulation as adhering to a certain standard of care that is uniform. I don't see it as protection for mothers and babies. I feel like the work that we do is very, very safe. It's much safer than what a lot of doctors do. Their attitude is different. It's been a six-year struggle to keep from being regulated out of our practice. This year we will be going back to the legislature and saying, "This bill's not working. We want a midwifery board. We want licensure and not just registration or certification through the health department. We want to be out of Health and Social Services and into Occupational Licensing, so that we have our own board through Occupational Licensing." When we got the bill in 1985, we had asked for that, but the governor had said no to the condition, so we changed it. At that point the Alaska Medical Association was trying to outlaw midwifery. We needed to get something passed, and we did get something passed very quickly. We realize now what we gave up. It's not working. We have to go back, and we have to say, "This is the history of it and it hasn't worked. This is what we need." I think we have a better chance of doing that with this administration. [Legislation was successfully passed in 1992 after this interview took place.]

One of the regulations that they're trying to put in Alaska is that you

have to be within twenty minutes of a hospital. That would eliminate most of Alaska. I will practice wherever I am if there's a need. I feel that it is a calling, not a job. It's the right thing to do. My heart goes out to women practicing where it's not legal, because they're so brave. But I would do it.

Spending time with my family is really important, and I've learned to draw a line and not let my practice take over my life. If it's evening or weekend time then it is family time. Aside from teaching a childbirth class one night a week, I don't see clients in the evening unless it is a postpartum home visit that I need to do right after a birth. I try to do those things during the daytime when my family is at work and at school. If someone calls me in the evening, I ask if I can call them back the next day instead of talking during dinner, which I used to do.

Midwifery is also physically grueling—sometimes my body doesn't stand up. I see an acupressurist once a week because I have to do things for myself. I also exercise and have a strong support system.

I have a lot of faith in birth even when there is fear. After a birth where there is a complication or problem and I'm back at home, I think about what's happened and wonder what if this would have gone differently? But I have a tremendous amount of faith when I'm at a birth that there's a higher power there with me. I usually think of me as more than one—the guides are there. I don't usually think of the fear when I'm at a birth. Sometimes I get a rush of fear, and I have to distinguish where it's coming from. Sometimes it might be coming from someone in the room—the husband or the woman, or from me. And then I use prayer—I guess you would call it prayer, meditation—just letting go and saying, "Okay, whatever, just let me know what it is I need to do." It works, it works really well.

I couldn't do midwifery if I didn't think there was a higher purpose to what I am doing. It's very difficult work, because you are putting yourself out there for everyone that you work with. You're taking on a lot of responsibility, and so are the women that I'm working with. I make sure that they do understand the responsibility. I'm not there to do it for them, I'm there to empower them to do it themselves. I feel like that is my work. I don't necessarily feel like my work is delivering babies as much as it is empowering women to give birth to their baby. I'm there to guide them. I think a lot of my work takes place during prenatal care counseling, when I work with women to accept the responsibility for their diet and their exercise. Just believing in their bodies is what they really need to give birth, that's the majority of the work. Then when it comes to the birth, if they have that, they can do it.

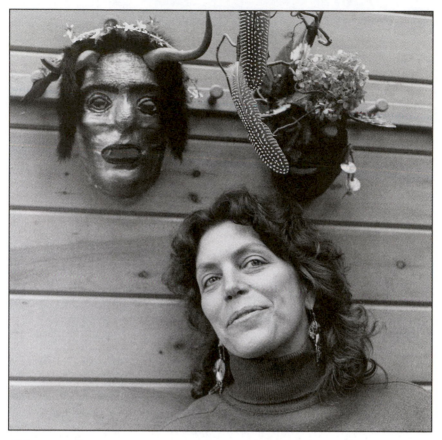

Carol Leonard

Carol Leonard is a New Hampshire certified midwife who was instrumental in the passage of legislation that allows midwives to practice legally in New Hampshire. She co-founded the Concord Midwifery Service and had attended over one thousand births before she stopped practicing in 1987. She was president of the New Hampshire Midwives Association from 1976 to 1985. One of the founding mothers of MANA, she served as president in 1986. In 1984, she was sent to the Congress of the International Confederation of Midwives, in Sydney, Australia, to represent MANA in the successful bid to have MANA included in the ICM membership. While she was there she was awarded a Bronze Medal for Bravery from the Australian government for saving a crashed hang glider pilot's life by performing CPR.

Carol stopped practicing midwifery when her husband, an obstetrician, died. She now consults and gives lectures on midwifery and is an avid herbalist, raising medicinal herbs with a current focus on herbs for the menopause years. She is a bodywork practitioner and uses polarity therapy and energy work combined with shamanic journeying as means of healing for those with chronic and terminal illness. She teaches a course called "Woman's Ordinary Magic," and a workshop called "Witches, Midwives, and other Healers." Carol has traveled to Russia, where she worked to improve maternity care, an effort that was highlighted on the TV show *20/20*. Carol has coauthored a book with Elizabeth Davis titled *Women's Wheel of Life: Thirteen Archetypes of Woman at Her Fullest Power* (1996).

Carol Leonard

I wanted to tell you my personal birth story because that is what actually got me started in midwifery. When I got to the hospital, I was contracting every minute and was eight centimeters dilated. But in the next three hours they did the whole schmiel as far as shave, enema, and then I was left alone in the bathroom for forty-five minutes. They told me to stop pushing while moving me into the delivery room, but I was bellowing like a moose in heat.

When my son Milan's head was crowning [stretching of the vaginal opening as the baby's head appears], I was burning like hell, so I put my hands down there and the doctor slapped my hand, tied my hands down, and said that I had contaminated his sterile field. He was treating me like an animal, I was shocked and I said, "Oh? My crotch wasn't sterile when I came in here."

I was so in love with my body and completely fascinated with the whole process of childbirth. I had done so well with no drugs and at the same time I had to deal with these maniacs . . . but you can't be mad when you're trying to have a baby. Afterward I looked at myself in the delivery room mirror and saw that I was shaved and cut and I looked like a trussed turkey. I said "Give me my baby right now," and they completely ignored me. I said, "Give me my baby NOW!" and they looked at me like I was postpartum psychotic already. The obstetrician flopped Milan on my chest, but my hands were still tied down. I didn't have any plans to be a midwife, but I knew then that I wanted to help women know about sane childbirth.

Three months later I went to my first birth with a general practitioner. After the first birth, when I was cleaning up I felt like I had always done it, like I had done it a thousand times and I knew exactly what to do. It was the most incredible feeling of rightness—"Hey, I'm back." The next birth I had been with the woman for twenty-four hours and the doctor was in the office and I called him when it got close. She was pushing and he was fussing around in her vagina and every time he fussed around she'd pull away. So I pushed his hand aside, and suddenly there I was with the baby being born. The next day I went over to humbly apologize for interfering, and he said, "Are you kidding? That was so beautiful. It made me realize that women should attend women." He never delivered another baby after that, but he loved to watch and was the greatest teacher. He taught me suturing and the old art of obstetrics—he always knew exactly what position the baby was in—the passenger and the passages [the baby as passenger, and the pelvis with its bony landmarks as the passages].

I'm really concerned that this apprenticeship model through which I learned midwifery is threatened and is going to be a dinosaur if people keep letting it go and giving it up. I will fight to the death for that kind of training because I feel that hands-on teaching is superior to institutional training. My dream is to have midwifery education accessible to women through their community colleges.

I am not attending births right now but doing what I call plain old-fashioned healing, bodywork with those who are dying. In the ancient way, the midwives brought in the babies and also laid out the dead as part of their role—from womb to tomb. A lot of what has happened to me is because of my husband Ken's death. His death stripped me of all my labels, everything that had been part of my life—my security, my definition of myself—my ego was pulled out from under me; even my dog ran away. His death was such a shock that I didn't speak for a whole year. I lived out in the woods and stayed in my right brain for the entire time. I didn't call myself a midwife anymore because I wasn't. I needed to take care of myself, but it never felt desolate or desperate or sad. It was a magical time. I spent a lot of time with the animals in the woods. My dog, Boar Woman, came then, and when I went into a deep trance, she would raise her leg and mark in a circle all around me like a guardian.

But I have to go back to the way Ken died. He had a long history of being a manic-depressive, and one day they called from work because he wasn't there. I knew there was something terribly wrong. He was an obstetri-

cian, and he hadn't missed a day in twenty-three years. I called the police then. The next day I got his letter in the mail and it was a beautiful love letter, and basically he said that he loved me more than I would ever know but that he was done. It wasn't out of anger or desperation but just that he felt like he had finished his work. The next page was this list of all his insurance policies, etcetera. That night I sat with my mother and I said to her, "Ken and I were so close, so psychically connected that I would know if he was dead, but he isn't dead yet."

The next morning I woke up and a pileated woodpecker that was on a tree, hopping around, and I was mesmerized. Then I thought, "What am I doing? My husband's missing!" So I went to his office to make sure everything was okay and they were still catching the babies. I came back and stood in the kitchen where it was real warm and sunny and quiet. There was a picture in the bathroom of him as a boy. It fell off the bathroom wall and hit the slate floor and the glass flew everywhere. My mother came down and said, horrified, "I hope that's not a bad sign." I said, "It is. He's dead. I need for you to leave right now."

I was on autopilot then. I went upstairs and took all my clothes off and anointed myself with rain oil that he loved and stepped out onto the balcony. The sun was really bright, hypnotic, white light, and absolutely still. And I heard him say "Carol," clear and soft. I wasn't hysterical; I wasn't hallucinating. And the way he said it, said it all: "I'm okay," very calm and reassuring.

And I said, "I don't understand. But I love you and I let you go." And when I said that, I felt him physically leave me. And a swirl of snow went down the field and down to the path to where he was, but I didn't know that. And I said goodbye. I went and laid down on my bed and waited. Fifteen minutes later my neighbor called and said that they were bringing a body from the tree by the path. The tree was our place, we called it "The Mother," and was where we went to meditate or when we needed to sort things out. So in what seemed like such a violent act, it felt to me that he went back to The Mother, the source. I honored his decision to do that, and so it has always felt that the way he left was sweet actually, so that I would know he was okay. That is what started the transformation for me, the crossover to do this kind of work. I was wide open.

Now I teach a course of woman's ordinary magic for accessing states of nonordinary reality and reviving the ancient art of "woman craft." Basically what it teaches is a trance technique to get people into their right brain, so they can tap this great landscape we have available to us, so much informa-

tion. Because we've been told that it doesn't exist, we totally shut it out. It's great to give women these tools so they can journey and find their guides and their messages. I've been using this with people who are acutely ill, because you tap into your own power, your power to heal yourself. Once you find those messages and those guides or allies, then you can get into personal healing.

I've recently returned from Russia, where I attended births with another American midwife. The first baby I assisted out is touted to be the first Russian baby to be delivered by an American. It was quite an honor—the parents named the boy after my son Milan. The video footage that we shot there was eventually used on *20/20*'s exposé of barbaric birth practices in the former Soviet Union. We were fortunate to get hooked up with a woman gynecologist who was the head ob/gyn at the clinic we were visiting. It was funny because she didn't speak a word of English and we didn't speak Russian, so the three of us spoke German. She introduced us to the head doctors at the rodoms, the Russian maternity houses, where Americans have never been. We filmed everything. They wanted us to film, because I think that the doctors know that the conditions are terrible; they wanted us to see it. We stood by and filmed a lot of their births. They wanted to see us work since we had been giving lectures and I had brought over videos of active births, like "Homebirth in Holland."

There is no contraception available in Russia, and an average Soviet woman has approximately fifteen abortions. The Soviet government thinks that the pill is harmful, and sees abortions as "cleansing." Women are left alone afterward to suffer, and the women are still made to feel guilty. The Soviet government is encouraging women to have more children, but the women don't want to bring children into the world without having food available. The doctors themselves are wonderful; they know the conditions are terrible, and when we were there they were eager to learn and see how we did births.

Women are mandated to have their babies in only one hour. They use five ampules of ergotrate straight IV push [a drug given intravenously that stimulates the uterus to have stronger contractions and can cause uterine rupture]. It is a slaughter! Their infant mortality rate is high, but their infant morbidity rate is really high! I didn't see many babies born with an Apgar over five [a rating of the condition of the newborn on a scale of one to ten; five and under indicates a baby in distress]; they are all cyanotic [deprived of oxygen] from the ergotrate, plus they use fundal pressure [pushing on the

uterus] for second stage [pushing stage]—they only allow the baby to be on the perineum for ten minutes. And the more I thought about it, the baby *does* need to be born in ten minutes with that much ergotrate and morphine. A woman we saw had three broken ribs; the doctors physically squeeze the babies out of these women. It's horrendous. It is an obsession with conformity, and everyone gives birth like a machine. Women seem to be a dispensable commodity. And then, after all that the women don't see their babies again for three to five days!

We were giving a lecture for some doctors when I heard a woman pushing down the hall, and I asked the doctor, "Is she in labor?" and he said, "She tries." So, with the next contraction I really heard her pushing, which was unusual since all the Soviet women were drugged with a morphine derivative—I don't know what it was but they all stared at the wall and didn't make one sound, not a peep. In the labor ward I thought they were all in early labor, but they were all almost ready to deliver but they still just stared at the wall. So I said to my partner, "You keep talking and I'll go check on this woman." I walked down the hall and into a labor room where this woman was completely alone. The great thing was that since all the doctors were at the lecture, she hadn't been medicated yet, she didn't have an IV [intravenous hookup]. She hadn't had any drugs, and *that* was why she was making noise. It was her first baby, she was a young Cossack woman. I just sat down next to her and started rubbing her back, and she folded into me. I was holding her and rocking her and the doctors all came running in and were shocked that I was touching her. They asked me if I wanted to do the birth. And I said, "Sure, just don't give her any medication." They said, "Well, she's not prepared," and I said, "No kidding" (they don't have prenatal childbirth classes there). And then a doctor told me that Soviet women didn't want to see their babies when they were born, and I thought, I don't think this woman is different from any other woman in the world. I said I think it will work out, and it did. It was a really nice testimony to the bonding process to watch this woman who was not prepared, and who was very shocked when the baby was brought up to her chest, unfold as she got to know her baby. The doctors were so shocked when we got the baby nursing; they said they couldn't sleep all night—they had never seen a baby nurse right at birth because the babies and women are usually so narcotized.

In the end, all it is, is changing attitudes about women and recognizing that they can give birth without all this routine stuff that they do now. That's actually the hardest thing for those in power to do—is just to love their

women and trust. Over there health care is not a priority; doctors are not revered. Military might is the objective.

They need midwifery care in Russia and to have active, unmedicated birth, respecting the woman's ability to give birth naturally. They need more than anything to learn how to love their women. The last thing they need is more technology—they've already taken what they've learned from the frightening German operating theaters of the twenties and thirties. What they need is to change their attitudes about women and not see them as machines and dispensable commodities. Women need to be loved and supported and empowered to give birth without all the drugs and technology. It doesn't even cost a lot of money, only love.

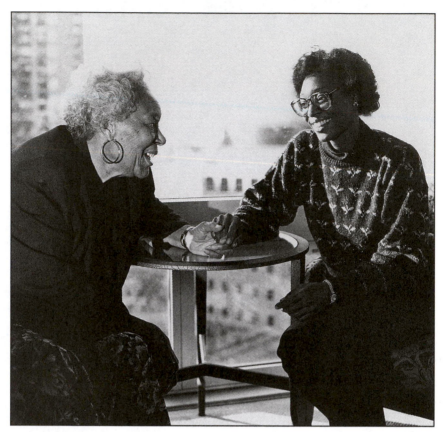

Gladys Milton

Gladys Milton lives in the panhandle of Florida, and over her many years of working as a midwife has attended births in Florida and in southern, rural Alabama. She received her midwifery license in 1959, and thirty years later she was asked to give it up by the Florida Department of Public Health, as they wanted to retire all the midwives. The midwifery supporters in Florida rallied and successfully won her battle in court, and Gladys still practices today in a birth center. Gladys's determination can be seen through her rebuilding (with her community's help) two birth centers that burned down. Her daughter (sitting with Gladys in her portrait) has also become a midwife. In 1976, Gladys was given the Sage Femme Award from MANA, and in 1992 she received the Woman of the Year Award. Many other awards acknowledge her service as a midwife. Gladys is a deacon and adult Sunday school teacher in her missionary Baptist church. Her goals and ambitions are to continue in midwifery, to expand her clinic, to make at least one new friend daily, to maintain old friendships, and to give and receive all the beauty that she possibly can each day.

Gladys Milton

When I got that award [Sage Femme Award from MANA], I loved hearing these words. Usually somebody come up and say all those nice things about you, when you're gone, and everybody that can hear something but you, you lying up there. Speak kind words to me while I can hear. I'm glad I was able to maintain the tears.

With every second Sunday in August we have homecoming for the clinic. All the children that were born there at the clinic want to come back and pay their respect to the clinic and talk to me and hug my neck. After seventeen years in the field, they're growing. I say, "All my babies are successful. As long as you're doing what you want to do, and doing a good job." Success isn't determined by the amount of energy you put out, real success is the amount of what you like that you can share.

I started in midwifery when I was somewhere about eight and ten years old. My mother's sister started out to be a midwife. Time dragged on; she delivered maybe five, six with no problem. Everybody had children before and they just had an easy delivery. Then she got a hold of one that was kicking and screaming and being all like that. Being new she didn't know what else to do. She just decided she would give up. And she did, even with everybody begging her, with empty pockets and everything to keep on. At this time she wasn't, I would say, more than twenty-four, when I was eighteen years old. This was during the depression years, thirty-two to thirty-four.

The granny midwives told us that they had the baby in that black bag. I

found that kind of hard to believe. As I grew a little older I noticed, Why she loosed all this big stomach. If the baby's in the bag, then why all of a sudden she got this stomach? I was still trying to figure out the birds and the bees and everything. Finally, I couldn't figure out intercourse. I thought that having intercourse made you have to wear Kotex. I had it all figured out backwards. That man surely want to know where he can have intercourse with a woman, that's what made her bleed. She had intercourse until she had to put on a Kotex.

My aunt never had any children. My aunt didn't know much more about babies than I did, other than her midwifery training. We had a real old trunk. That was a great big one. All the secrets got put in there and all that kind of stuff. I watched good where they kept the key—there in the hall? buried in the papers? or in there? I liked fishing. But if I could, I was not going to go fishing with her, because I was going to get the key when she gets out of sight and get in that trunk, and get that book and read it. She had the midwife's manual, remnants of her packs and stuff. I wanted to get that manual. And I would get it and I would read, and figure out about babies. Then I saw scissors and all these things in the pack. Different things. What they going to need these scissors for? I sure don't see any thread or needles here or nothing. What they need the scissors for? I just don't know. I couldn't figure that out, but I read that, and then I got a little wiser. I figured out that actually this woman does have a baby. I thought this is the most impossible thing in the world. There is no way the woman can get no baby born in the world, unless they're gonna cut it out with the scissors.

Then I went to this meeting that turned out to be a prenatal care meeting. The nurses would come and do them. This one nurse, Nurse Thelma Hessler, that's her name, she conducted that meeting that night. At the end of the meeting she said, "Any of you I can train to be a midwife?" I was the first one to say, "I sure don't." When I got home, I told my son about it. Then I start thinking so serious about it. I talked to a very nice minister friend of mine, and I said that I didn't specially want to go, 'cause I was always going to be on the winning side and the winning side is not midwifery, not even until today, thirty-two years later. It's not the winning side for a lot of people. When I was a child I wanted to play ball on the side I thought was going to win. I played sorry and anybody, but I was gonna get on the team that was gonna win. So I said, "Oh, Lord what is this?" and I thought about it everywhere I went. Funny, if I were to lay down at night, I'd be thinking about it. I went in, "You got anything you're gonna do more important than

that?" and I say, "Yes!" He said, "What?" Well, I couldn't think of what. I say, "Oh, a lot of things," and I went on to my room and I went to bed. In that bed there was that little voice. Days and days and days and days, when I settled down I couldn't think of anything else, that little voice would cut in on it. I finally got sick of that little voice. And the little voice saying it'll take my hand off. I hear the little voice again. Then it came time to go down to the clinic, where I saw her. Started over to her two or three times. Finally something showed me over to where she was in a line giving children shots. Finally I said, "Miss Hessler?" She said, "What is it?" and I said, "I want to, what we were talking about." See that was her way of asking me. Everybody gave her such a cool reception, I said, "Whenever you get time some time, you think about this." She said, "Wait a minute. I got time right now." She didn't let me go. She said, "Stand right there." She went and got a nurse to replace her in the shot line. We ended up in a little conference room, and within, I'll say, thirty minutes she contacted the state of Florida. Because you see by this time all the older midwives that I knew, they were getting too old to practice. A lot of them had died.

Within the hour all of my arrangements were made and we went over to meet the two doctors. One of them was . . . I forget . . . oh, Dr. Mathews and Dr. O'Neil. This was right following World War II. They were service doctors. They had come to our little town. We only had two doctors in the little town. It was Dr. Young and Dr. Holly. Dr. Young had died; there was only Dr. Holly in the whole town, three or four little town area. They came from the service there. They came to supplement doctors there, where they were going to go to a small place because they're needed. You know that's just what happens to little towns like ours. They come and they work and they get all their education money paid and everything and they lift up and go over there somewhere and join up where they can make some money. Anyway, they came, and Nurse Hessler had took me over.

I'm a blabbermouth and I have a whole lot of friends. My daughter tells me sometimes, "Say, that's just your way right around here." I also let her know that I don't have any race problem with their business. A lot of racial problems in our area. There still is . . . colors, religions, and all that stuff. Through the years I have seen my practice flow from indigent white and black to middle-class white. Mostly my practice is, I'd say about nine-to-one middle-class white. We counted it up ourself. One hundred and ninety four births and we only had three blacks among them.

But back then, we went on and up and got my training complete there.

A lot of brochures and a nurse came up and help me get my pack together. Had an old sewing machine—she had me to get some ninety-inch un-bleached muslin and then take it to the laundry get it washed, and for her all the things have to be precise. She came up and helped me cut up the whole pack and showed me how to sterilize it. I sterilized my first pack in a pressure cooker under twenty pounds of pressure, now we use an autoclave, but at that time we just had the pressure cooker.

I had to observe, then do, either twenty-five or fifty births, it's been so long. Then they let me do twenty-six—that's all that was required of me, and a written test. Started out work in October fifty-nine.

These were all homebirths. I wasn't doing so many, but I managed to make it. We talking about on the road. We talking about getting up about two o'clock in the morning, twenty-five miles down to Crestview. I would have been steering and most of the births were between one and five [in the morning]—there was a gospel program on. Anyway, it's from the station in Maxwell, Tennessee. They played a lot of gospel music, and I'd be riding to those places keeping time with the music in my foot, trying to get there in time. I drived fast. I never got any arrests for speeding. If I got to go any-where, and I got some open road, I'm going. Sometime they used to, this was later on, get on the CB and say, "All right Gladys, slow down, you're just going too fast." I was twenty-two miles from the clinic, even since I had the clinic. I CB them and tell them, "Hey, get down there on the corner and help me get on through town. I'm in a hurry." They get down there.

My only requirement then was to go to the house and get familiar with the house and see how do you live, and get to know them a little bit and more or less learn the way, 'cause you get a call at three o'clock in the morning, how else you gonna know where it is? I always knew where it was, and if I was getting there say, "Meet me at Old North Creek church," sayin', "There will be a black truck waiting there for you to show you the way." I would have been scared, but I don't have sense enough to be scared. The roads, they were not paved then. I'm not such a good driver when it come down to staying out of ditches and that kind of stuff, but I have never been stuck going on my way to one of my babies.

Like I say, I'm from that they call the Bible Belt down there. I'm not ashamed to say that I pray before every birth. Ask the Lord to give us, if it's his will, give us a safe birth and also give me the insight to know in time if I need to ship it out. So I go off to the bathroom—but not for the regular thing [reason] that we go. I go in there and communicate with my Creator.

To see if there is something I ought to see. He'll give me the assurance that everything is all right. One girl I went right back in and I said this was her first baby, and she was dragging along a little bit. I'm not very happy taking first baby. I take 'em by size and this was a little bitty girl, usually smaller than I take 'em. If you take some big person like me, I'd be deformed to have a small pelvis. Everything else is big and adequate about us, so the pelvis most likely is too. But this was a little bitty girl. She went and kind of pushed a little bit, but I didn't seem to get any responses I wanted to get. So I went to the bathroom. I went in there and stayed there a while, and came back. The Lord says everything is all right, don't need to go anywhere. I'll tell 'em if I need to go, and then I'll ask their opinion. "Are you satisfied staying here? As far as I can see there's no problem, but would you be happier if I took you to the hospital," and most of them are not. I told her, I said, "Ceciel, the Lord says that if you push a little bit more, you'll get your baby." So she did. She pushed a little bit more and here come a baby, a big boy.

When they abolished us, I say licensed midwives, we don't like lay mid-wives—lay seems inferior, not trained or something to mean, anyway we fought 'til they took that off our name in Florida. Lay midwives, I don't mind being called a licensed midwife, because that's what I am, but I'm not any lay. We were successful in getting that taken off our name. I think it's a matter of educating a lot of people. People don't know what we do.

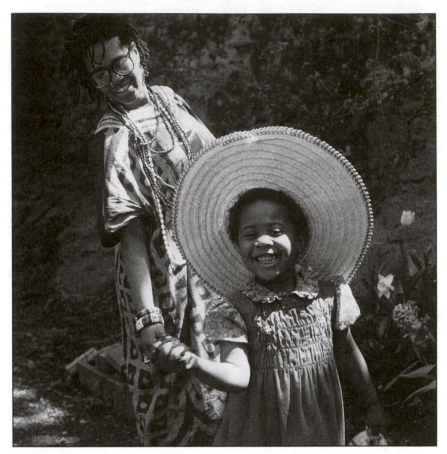

Shafia Munroe

Shafia Munroe was born in Alabama, where her great-aunt was a well-known midwife. Midwives from Africa and the West Indies were Shafia's first teachers. At the age of twenty-one, she had her first baby at home with a white male doctor; her five subsequent children were delivered with midwives. She has been involved with public health politics in Boston, a city where the infant mortality rate is third highest in the nation. She is the founder of the Traditional Childbearing Group in Boston, an organization that teaches African-American perspectives in childbearing, as well as breastfeeding and labor support. It also provides prenatal care to help women care for themselves and their unborn children given the stresses of poverty and racial inequality. Shafia now lives in Portland, Oregon, where she started the International Center for Traditional Childbearing.

Shafia Munroe

All religions have a high regard for the midwife. Midwives in Africa did marriage counseling, helped to wrap the dead, worked with herbs, and did abortions. The Africans look at it as a valued job. My midwifery is based on an African perspective, which I see as one way to bring people back to knowing that we had a culture where our babies were healthy. In Africa they haven't gone through the witch burning, and midwives are still honored. When I asked my friend from Senegal, who has attended five thousand births, why she became a midwife, she said: "When I was little, I used to see this person coming into a crowd, and there would be a break, an opening for her, and I would say, 'Who is this person?' And they told me, 'She is the midwife who caught all the babies.' I saw the respect, and how she loved everyone."

My father told me about my great-aunt, who was a midwife, but I never met her. But my grandmother, who is still alive at one hundred years old—she went to births and I got to talk to her a lot about midwifery, and breastfeeding, and voodoo, and food and herbs that the Africans brought off the boats as slaves.

I use a southern tradition and an African tradition, and both of them change a bit as they are used again and again. For example, when the little baby gets the hiccups you take the string off the baby's clothes, put it in your mouth and put it over the soft spot [the space remaining in the still-soft skull of an infant]; this is a southern tradition, and they do the same thing in Africa

New statistics from public health show that the Hispanics are doing as

well as white Americans [in terms of infant mortality], who are doing as well as the Europeans; the blacks are the lowest. African Americans were brought here against their will in slavery. The anger of black Americans is generational, it's genetic. It's anger from Africa when you saw your husband taken away. I'm angry. I've got two fibroids [benign tumor made up of fibrous and muscular tissue in the uterine wall]—it happens a lot to African women who live in industrial countries and are under a lot of stress. It's very prominent in our race.

I was raised in a spiritual family. My father was very religious. When I was fifteen, I became a Muslim. When I was little, anything that needed help I wanted to help it—a sick puppy, a rabbit. I was praying over the puppy and running downstairs in the middle of the night to feed the puppy—it was kind of like midwifery.

When my mother died, we moved with my father to another woman's house who was pregnant. I just loved her stomach, and I would hang out under her belly. She said, "Shafia, you are so interested, you should become an obstetrician." My father said, "Why not be a midwife? Your great-aunt was a midwife."

Whenever I go to a delivery, I usually try to take a shower for cleanliness, but also because for a Muslim water has a special meaning, it's called a *gushina:* you are washing things away from you. And then I make a special prayer before I leave the house that Mosha, the Creator, will show me something that I haven't seen. In the South, when the midwife first came to the house, we all got down on our hands and knees and held hands and prayed. The midwife didn't just go in and take a blood pressure. I like that. I tell people before the birth that I might pray out loud. I pray in Arabic. There is a certain chapter in the Koran that is for complicated births, so I'm working on memorizing that. It's important to pray at easy births too. I try to be humble and not attribute success of a birth to myself, but first to God, and then the family, and not get into the ego thing of how I helped you to have your baby. But I'm just there as an aid to the natural process.

There's an important ritual of talking to the pregnant woman to see how she's doing. I can't walk into someone's house after the birth where there is no food, or no food cooked, the house is a wreck, the baby is in her arms crying, they've got tears, the kids are watching something on the TV they shouldn't be—I can't go in and think, Yep, blood pressure is fine, uterus is shrinking, I'll be back tomorrow. I can't do that.

An African friend of mine cried after her birth in the hospital and said,

"Shafia, I can't believe it—if I was in my country I'd have people here and visitors. My mother would bathe me in sea water, and have me stand over steam to get the clots out [from the uterus so it will contract and not bleed] and massage my breasts." It's the care we want, not our blood pressures taken. I cook a nice peanut stew from West Africa. When a baby is born you want to put wetness back into the mother, and I used to always make a pot and bring it back to the mother on the first day after the birth. I used to wrap the mother's stomach and give the baby her first bath, or help the mother with a postpartum bath of herbs. After having my babies at home, I loved the midwife giving my baby her first bath. It's so nurturing.

Midwifery is the most important thing in my life after God. It's like being on a mission, on a journey; I'm being compelled. It's been a struggle with my husbands—I've been married a few times. It's hard having it more important than them. But I've been with this brother ["man" in African American slang] for thirteen years; he's a very nice husband. He loves children, more than I do. But I get more enjoyment from knowing the women and making a difference in their lives. Some midwives love children, but I love women. You work with a woman for nine months. Someone would say to me, "You'd like to start a day care?" And I say, "That's not it." I love women. I love to see them happy and at peace so that they can raise their children.

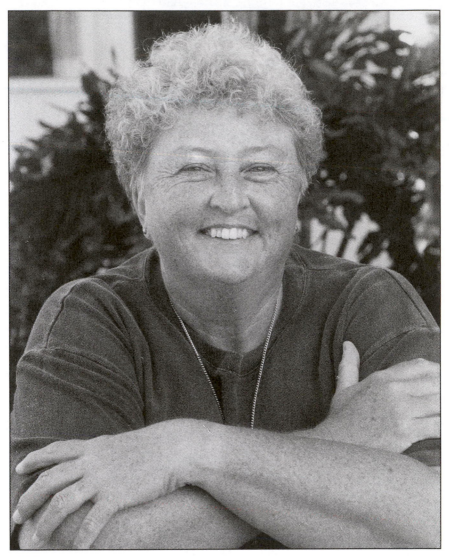

Sister Angela Murdaugh

A graduate of Columbia University in New York, Sister Angela Murdaugh has been a nurse-midwife for the past twenty-three years. She started one of the first freestanding birth centers in the country in Raymondville, Texas (near the Mexican border), in conjunction with a migrant worker health clinic. She has long been active in midwifery organizations. In 1981 she became president of the ACNM, serving a two-year term, and she conceived and facilitated the birth of MANA. It was by her invitation in 1981 that midwives of diverse backgrounds from all over North America came to join in a discussion of lay and nurse-midwifery. She has been active in the National Association of Childbearing Centers (NACC) and has taught clinical skills and served as a mentor to many nurse-midwifery students. She currently runs a freestanding birth center, Holy Family Services, in Weslaco, Texas, where she provides affordable and respectful care to underserved and impoverished women.

Sister Angela Murdaugh

I've been a nun for thirty-one years. My order is all health care people, so midwifery wasn't a strange career for me to enter. We have our own place outside of town on four-and-a-half acres, and we live there, too. The church lets us use the land and sponsors us so we can be nonprofit to receive grants, but they put very little money in it. If you are at Holy Family you have to want to live a simple lifestyle, live in a community, really care about the people around you, not live an isolated life, or you won't last.

The way we built the birth center with flowers and animals came from living on a small piece of property. As well as being witness to a simple life-style, we produce some of our food and are tuned in to the earth. We have air conditioning for the families, but the patients often ask for it to be turned off. We live without it, and it makes you appreciate the shade trees, little breezes, and cooling off at night.

Being a nun and having religious faith certainly made me able to stay where I am and do what I had to do, because I didn't have to be reimbursed. I live a simple lifestyle. I feel happy about what I do because I was called to do that—it's how I'm supposed to serve God. Some of it isn't so much my part, my free choice, but how God can work in the world through me, and come to some realization of that. You see miracles happen in your hands and you become faith-filled. You know *you* didn't do it. Your hands moved, but something else did that. That's the perspective it's brought to me that's been fulfilling for my spiritual, emotional, psychological life.

I call the difficult births "three Hail Mary deliveries"—yes, definitely you have faith to fall back on. Plus, I live in community with other sisters who have been really supportive. When I was young I lived with two older sisters who were like other mothers or my midwives. They took care of me. There's a lot of strength in living with people who are aimed at the same thing you are. Life is difficult, with so many bumps. It's nice somebody's not on the bump when you are. Right now we're living *and* working at the birth center, so we're not divergent. There are nine sisters and three volunteer nurses ministering to those poor people. We have a kitchen and living room with a big screened patio, two wings with five bedrooms and two or three bathrooms each. Behind that there's a building with bedrooms and a quiet room for reading and writing, and then we have a chapel between us and the birth center. In the center there are birth units, the office, and a classroom.

Most of my clinical practice has been in south Texas. It's very Spanish, one of the ten poorest counties in the United States, per capita income is low, 20 percent unemployment. We have tourism (beach, old folks) or agriculture. I love the Mexican influence, their compliance during maternity care. The biggest things in life to them are children and land—where ours are money, moving ahead, prestige. They are gentle, want to please, and aren't ambitious. I find it hard to take care of people who are not poor. I'm not used to it, the demands. When I was president of the American College of Nurse-Midwives I lived in Washington, D.C., and took call [was on call] for some homebirth nurse-midwife services. I used to laugh at some of the calls in the middle of the night that could have *positively* waited until morning.

We do about 350 births a year. Our people migrate to do farmwork here in the winter. I believe the way they give birth is affected by their relation with the land and agriculture, although they wouldn't be able to articulate that. It's such a wonderful expectation they have, to be producing life. They're willing to do what it takes to have it. Urban women don't have that. Just living on a piece of land, growing a few flowers gives you a little more control over your life.

My hardest challenge as a midwife is to be a person who's very organized and yet be forced to live a life of always being in a state of readiness, and prepared for the unexpected, and not being able to plan for that. It's become real frustrating not only in regard to having enough staff to keep the birth center covered, but to have enough time for myself. People say "take time," but there's no *taking* time. It has to be provided. Lack of freedom to come and go as you please. I have a sense of responsibility—these are poor people,

and I'm not taking that lightly. But then I got to know more midwives, so I have a fair number I can call now for help or a break. When I was younger I felt so tied to my job. Now I can plan for those chances to re-create myself. Praise God I'm not one who needs constant stimulation. One good trip every few months. I find lecturing really revitalizing. I just did the Midwifery Today conference. It's ego-stimulating, boosts you up, this work is worthwhile. I'm not afraid to go in cold and have people ask questions, because I have a good basic body of knowledge from my own experience.

I've been real fortunate with physicians. I've been free all my life to shake the dust off, to not put up with them—that's been real painful for some people. I didn't try to get hospital privileges. There was a time when hospital privileges didn't work out, and I just said fine.

Life is unpredictable. You can't plan. I've learned to say my little prayer. When I used to have a primip [woman having her first baby] hanging out at the birth center, I never could go to sleep. Now I say it's time to rest, and I'm asleep before I know it. You learn not to fight it as time goes on.

So many wonderful things have happened because of midwifery. I had some miles on my frequent flyer and I wanted to go to Hawaii. There's a midwife in Hawaii I had done a favor for when she was a student, so I went to visit and they treated me like I was family, showed me around, and brought me into their homes. I've gotten back every bit as much as I've ever given. I'm not going to get a high place in heaven. My rewards are right here. The clinic where I started midwifery had its twenty-fifth anniversary. I went to the reception, and there were college kids from really poor agricultural families— a boy I delivered has his own child. It was heartwarming to receive the adulation of people who never forgot you as having been their *partera* [Spanish for midwife]. You couldn't forget these folks—like the lady who hemorrhaged after every child, and we were all prepared for it after the third—"I remember you!"

My sister once drove me down to the Rio Grande Valley to see the nurse-midwives in that area. We stopped at a gas station where I'd gone for eight-and-a-half years, and the man said something's wrong with my old beatup Pontiac station wagon, and he sent me across the street. So my sister and I sat there on two folding chairs with a fan, talked to his wife. The man went off to the junkyard and worked away. He presented us with a bill for eight dollars. "This can't be all!" I said. "You delivered two of my grand-children. We'll take care of it," he replied. That's the kind of stuff you see. They'll help you out, and they're happy to do that.

So I don't hesitate to ask. My services are valuable, and someone owes me for providing them. It's part of keeping dignity. We don't give free care—I won't give it. Outside of high risk, my only reason for throwing somebody off the caseload is if they think you'll do this for nothing. Our country has done that to poor people—let children grow up without a sense of responsibility. These are such wonderful people. We get some third-party reimbursement through Medicaid, but a lot of our clients pay out of pocket. They work in the yard for five dollars an hour, or clean, cook, sew, paint, contract. We barter for about 25 percent of the births. I have about 88 percent monetary recovery, much higher than doctors. I don't charge way more than something costs, so there's not a big profit motive. I can say, "If you don't pay, the people behind you aren't going to get it." I charge $1,000 now. I try to match Medicaid (with facility and professional fee together it's about $890). We give $100 off if they pay before the baby is born. About 10 percent want nurse-midwives or a birth center, and they can pay. If they have a third-party payer (about 4 percent of my practice) we have them pay $500 out of pocket and reimburse them if need be. I itemize their bills, and it usually runs about $1,800.

Personally, I'm getting older and have to slow down. I like administration, so I see myself spending more time on that. I'll stay in clinical work, although lately I've had another nurse-midwife at the birth center full-time.

I'm not good at writing, but I think I could write more than I do—mine would be a seasoned opinion. Speaking is my medium. I like to do conferences, and I volunteer to serve on committees more than I used to. I'm on the disciplinary committee for the ACNM. They need people with compassion and who have been around. I say it whenever I get the chance: "You should never, ever be afraid to write down what you did, or to show it to anybody else. If you're not doing what you should, be thankful that somebody will show you how to do it. Nobody expects you to be perfect, even the ones looking at you. You have to be ready to change."

One of my ten good qualities is that I am a good storyteller, and finally I have enough stories to tell. I've been in practice for twenty years, and I trade stories with other CNM's. One story will lead to another. Sometimes, when you are young, you have more guts. When you're older, you are more circumspect, even if you are more experienced. You mature in your profession as a woman. I tell stories with my students. It's a poignant way to teach. They pick up nuances by my relating experiences. It gets my point across. I try to help them understand you must treat each woman with respect and

friendship, but they will not be your friends. You may not remember them, or they you. This was a crossroads, a gift to you, but you were there just to meet their needs. Birth is a blip on the continuum of life. I'm providing expertise as a teacher, and you're actually paying me, but pregnancy and birth are your responsibility. I'm not going to police you. Enjoy midwifery, but it's not the end-all and be-all of your emotional fulfillment, just your professional fulfillment.

Different people have different psychological strengths. I've had partners fizzle or go on to do even bigger things. Extraneous things can cause burnout. Sacrifices are necessary. Being a midwife is stressful. Every day you're at work, making decisions. It's not rote. At some point, you need a break. Midwives get into foolish situations occasionally, like getting into practice by themselves.

I had a good neonatologist friend who once said, "Isn't it nice that we're finally at the age that everybody feels we have something to tell them?" You never stop being a student, but there's a point where your learning is so much more than anyone else's. When I first began, fetal monitoring was in an infantile state, no sonograms, doptones with incredible static [sonograms and doptones are two forms of ultrasound that enable one to see or hear a baby's heartbeat]. Out of a caseload of 250, it was not unusual for me to lose four stillborns a year. Now I rarely have one, because there's so much more we can know. The technology need not to be applied to every pregnancy, but we have so many more tools. My heart goes out to young midwives because the body of knowledge is so great today. You have so much to learn. The programs keep getting a little bit longer. Now there is herpes, HIV, chlamydia, monitor strips to read, etcetera. The understanding of Rh − [a factor in defining blood types; an incompatibility between mother and fetus can cause serious problems with the fetus] was just beginning, babies were transfused. NICUs [neonatal intensive-care units] have been developed since I became a midwife. We just used to keep preemies warm and put a feeding tube down.

I feel like I have made some national contributions to midwifery. I chose to be president of the ACNM and I worked on the joint statement between the ACOG [the American College of Obstetricians and Gynecologists] and the ACNM. I remember the president of the ACOG spouting off that there should be a statement that every woman should be seen by an obstetrician. I said, "Okay, if you make sure it happens, no matter how rural and isolated the women are, at no extra cost you'll go to them if need be, and

that your members may not refuse to see someone being seen by a nurse-midwife." He decided that perhaps such a statement was not necessary.

The ACNM convention the year I was president had the open-forum topic "Should nursing be a requirement as a background for lay midwifery?" and as usual we had a split. My subsequent efforts to get lay midwives and nurse-midwives together was probably the greatest thing I've done. I knew some people from NAPSAC [National Association of the Preservation of Safe Alternatives in Childbirth] where I had spoken, and some nurse-midwives who had been lay midwives prior to certifying. Some received it well, and some didn't. I was very naive about it—I thought nobody would mind if you talked. The group feeling was positive for almost everybody. I never expected it would go where it did [into the development of MANA as an organization]. I remember pleading for objective standards of education and practice in midwifery. Most of the time I was just an instrument as a catalyst for change with midwives. I had no axe to grind, and I am fair and just. I have my opinions, which has been an advantage. I'm compassionate. I know where people have been, that you shouldn't judge until you have all the evidence.

I *do* feel like I've changed the world. I believe I made a difference. I used to ask God: "Please, don't let me be called tonight, please let me sleep." At night now I pray, "God, all I ask, if You call me, is that You give me the strength to do it." I wouldn't do it if it wasn't making a difference, especially because I'm working with poor people. If my being there was one less dose of Demerol, if I was the narcotic for their personal strength, that is worth my being a midwife. We pass through this life to do good. Midwifery is my way of serving the world.

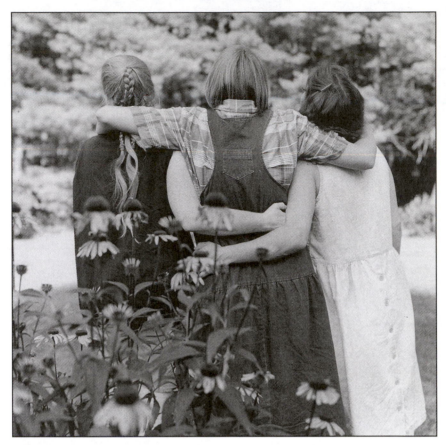

Anonymous Midwife

This midwife has been working in a state where her practice of midwifery is illegal. After her own home-birth experience, women in her community started asking her to be with them at their births. She felt like some help was better than no help at all, and so she began studying about birth through any workshop that came her way and through self-study with obstetric texts. After serving her community for eleven years, the pressure of working illegally has forced her to stop attending births—leaving women in her area without the choice of having attended homebirths. Some of these women are now birthing alone. She is accompanied in her portrait by her two apprentices; all three were pregnant and practicing at the time this photograph was taken.

Anonymous Midwife

I live in a hostile environment for homebirth and lay midwifery. I have for the most part felt like there isn't an out-and-out witch hunt, mostly because we've been careful to remain fairly invisible and not step on people's toes. But we did have a situation after a birth that went absolutely fine when a man from the health department tracked down the parents and tried to bully them into giving him information. He tracked down at least one other family and again told them lies as to what would happen to them if they didn't cooperate. What it made me realize was that although I have felt all along that they are not out there trying to find me, if we ever had a fetal or maternal death . . . It's an awful feeling to be blatantly breaking the law in this kind of work. You can just get an inkling of what the ramifications would be.

I make it real clear at the first visit and I say to my clients, "You need to understand that you can't refer to me as your midwife. I can only accept my fee in cash. Should we need to transport to the hospital, I would certainly share any pertinent information, but I would have to be referred to as your friend, so that there is no misunderstanding."

I used to be more reluctant to actually say that I'm breaking the law, but I'm not anymore since the experience of having the health department tracking people down made me realize that I didn't want to pussyfoot around the issue. One thing that has always been a concern for me is the question whether that fear would interfere with my judgment—like when it's time to

transport to the hospital from a homebirth. I've learned that it doesn't, so that's been a relief.

Somewhere in the state's agenda is [the desire to] somehow get rid of non–nurse-midwives. They've revised the rules and regs for nurse-midwifery and greatly enlarged the section on how to lose your license, including aiding and abetting a lay midwife, or providing secret medicines. They don't even address what a secret medicine is—I think it refers to herbs and homeopathy, which to them are secret. But the bottom line is that this is a hostile environment for homebirth. Not for midwifery—midwifery is growing within the medical establishment.

I see that more and more, that American midwifery is coming under the auspices of medicine, and for the masses of people out there that's great because it's the only way to get midwifery to them right now. So I'm not bemoaning that, but I shudder at the thought that this will be *the* definition of midwifery or midwife. The rise in CNMs is great, but I hope it doesn't change the definition of what a midwife is to be—the masculization of the midwife with the old reliance on medical training, medical procedures and protocol, and medical mindset. I really see medicine as we know it here in America as something very male. For me the standard definition is who I am as the traditional midwife. There are deviations from that which require prefixes—nurse-midwife, certified midwife, and you can alter that definition by whatever prefix you put on it. They are all fine, but I hate to think that we are going to alter that basic definition, because then we've lost the roots of all of it.

I have thought for years and years that midwives are handmaidens, service-oriented people, but I've always felt that they should be handmaidens to women and not to the system, and not to the establishment and not to doctors and medical schools, but their service should be to women. And that's not necessarily what I see happening in general.

All the things that first attracted me to this work are still there, and if it weren't for that, the rest of this would make it impossible. I see this work as a gift, to me, and also to the people that I work with. It's basically uplifting, and as the years go by, while more of the baggage is becoming visible, the driving force is positive and wonderful. You see a birth, and as most births unfold, you've watched magic, you've watched God, you've watched miracles, you've watched nature—you've seen it all! Right there before your eyes—and have been able to participate in it in a very special way. It comes with a price, but it's a pretty wonderful thing to walk around with.

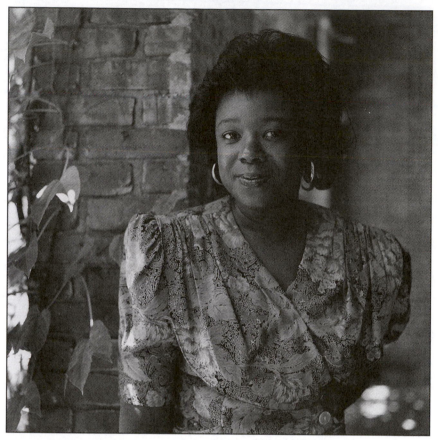

Jo-Anna Rorie

Jo-Anna Rorie is an assistant professor of public health at the Boston University School of Public Health. She is the former director of the ob/gyn services at the Dimmock Community Health Center in Roxbury, Massachusetts, and one of the founders of a home for drug-addicted pregnant women at this facility. A graduate of the Yale University Nurse-Midwifery Program, she also has a master's degree in public health from Harvard University. She is personally dedicated to the creation of a national public health policy for women and children. She presently lives in Dorchester, a neighborhood in Boston, with her mother. In a city where women of color are confronted by poverty and racism, her refusal to accept no as an answer to proposals for health care has led to the creation of essential and vital services for them.

Jo-Anna Rorie

If you were involved in the era of the civil rights movement, whether it was for Latinos, Hispanics, blacks, or women, you remember, as I do, how there was a fervor, an intensity and commitment, that, having experienced it, you never want to move away from, because it was good, because it was right. We were working toward a world that was going to be fair for everybody, toward being a country that was fair for everybody. And this conviction is seared in here, inside me. I don't wear an Afro and my hair has chemicals in it, I went to two Ivy League schools, but whatever I do, it is always done with the intention of a continuing commitment to improve conditions for the people in the community that I grew up in, the community that I know. And more particularly, that commitment means I never, never forget that I am an African-American woman, a midwife and health care administrator, working and surviving in a country driven by racism.

To this very day, people struggle to understand why black babies [in the United States] die at a higher rate than other babies do. And what I was struck most by at public health school is the fact that in all sorts of circumstances and stages of life, blacks die at a higher rate than whites. What is it that seems to kill black Americans before they are even born? I contend that it is the fact that our experience in this country was very, very different from that of other blacks on this earth because we were brought here as slaves and forced to serve as slaves. The chains were literally removed from our feet and hands and placed around our minds and hearts. And I believe that this histori-

cal experience is what kills us off so early in this country where we are not wanted, where we must struggle, we must fight forever for that piece of the American Dream promised to all. This is why our kids, these young blacks, shoot themselves and each other.

Given the fact of racism, the only way I got through a school of public health was by simply refusing to accept the fact that I was different because I'm black and knowing that any time I was confronted with racism I had to head it straight on, face it, and accept the reality that I may make people uncomfortable; I will talk to people in positions of great power this way. You have to say what you see, and you don't take no for an answer. You sometimes have to make people squirm.

At present, I am the primary provider for clients at the Houston House, a residential treatment program for pregnant and drug-addicted women who are also connected with the Department of Correction. It holds fifteen mothers and fifteen babies. The women at Houston House have relatively short sentences, about one year, for minor offenses, and they come early in their pregnancy and stay for nine months to a year, during which time they receive comprehensive care. It is an opportunity for most of these women to have a second chance at life and an opportunity to be the mothers they knew they could be. Many of them have long-term drug histories, and children who have been placed in the custody of the Department of Social Services. And we have had some really good success stories. At present, as the director of the ob/gyn services here at Dimmock Community Health Center, I have the authority and have been here long enough to have some say about deliveries and practices, to have colleagues say, "If this is the way Jo-Anna says it is, then this is accurate, this is so, this is true."

When I first set up a midwifery service, people didn't even know what a midwife was. Yes, you were a nurse, but then you were this thing called a midwife. People would say things to me like, "You're neither fish nor fowl." And it's true—I'm neither fish nor fowl; I'm a midwife. I've struggled hard with the system to have midwives empowered. At Beth Israel Hospital in Boston, I helped put together some very good protocols that are still utilized today. I worked very, very hard to become the director of ob/gyn services. And it's nice to now see how new midwives coming on staff don't have to struggle for the right to practice. They can write prescriptions, hospitals are welcoming them with their arms wide open, everyone's hiring midwives. There just aren't enough to go around! They are getting lucrative financial packages and their malpractice paid, and that's outstanding. But I know,

personally, that there was a price to pay for achieving this, and we paid it. We really paid it.

I think of myself as a midwife-teacher. I'm an aggressive manager in labor and delivery. I was trained at a high-risk center, and I learned first-rate technology at Yale and at Georgetown. But I learned to be a midwife on my own. And that part of my learning is inside me and connects me to other women, and that's what I draw on to know what is happening with my patients in labor even though I've had no children of my own. That is what let's me know when she's ready to push, or when she's too tired and needs a break, or I need to touch her or I need to walk with her or I need to talk with her—that piece I didn't learn at Yale. That is what I learned year after year after year sitting with and working with women in labor, talking with other midwives, just being with women. Now I don't know that you can get that in any educational program. I got my midwifery from working with women, watching women, and looking at women.

I used to expend about 80 percent of my emotional and psychological energy protecting myself and my patient from the system over the years. Happily, I don't do that quite so much anymore because people are now used to midwives being around. I'd be perfectly amenable to going to homebirths, but I deliver in the hospital because it's where my population goes. In spite of all our progress, I'm still always cognizant of the fact that I'm in the hospital and that we are still at a place where a midwifery mistake is a horrific mistake, while a medical mistake is just another medical mistake. If we have a bad outcome, it's really a *bad* outcome! And it may affect other midwives' practices also.

I see another part of my job, my life's purpose really, as an advocate for women's health issues and working toward a comprehensive health policy in this country for women and children. What I'd really like is to be the secretary of health on a national level. The problems change and the problems get bigger. Poverty gets worse. We simply do not have adequate and consistent public health policies in our country. Women are homeless in numbers that they never have been before, and women are using crack and cocaine in numbers that we have never seen before. Then HIV came along. . . . And I know that our educational programs never prepared us for this. And because the political atmosphere seems almost hostile to women and children, a lot of my energy goes toward advocacy and community teaching. I speak to groups to inform them about what is going on in terms of public health: where the money is and how it's being dispensed, or dispersed and not dispensed. I let

people know about the current house bills that might have an effect upon them.

People died for the right to vote and the right to speak, and too many women died before abortion was legalized, and we cannot be silent in the face of this. I talk to my community groups about how we need to attend public meetings, we need to be present, we need to be vocal, because if we don't we'll be right back where we started. We've had to adjust to the gag rule and not say the "A" [abortion] word at certain times. I get a call from a reporter asking, "So how are you going to respond to the gag rule?" and I say, "Are you kidding—under no circumstances, ever, is any bone in this body going to withhold information from a woman—never!"

Another important aspect to my thinking is my belief that technology is losing its flair so to speak and that it's time to give up health care practice dictated by the medical model, because it just doesn't work anymore. I'm not so sure it ever worked. We hoped that technology would lower the infant mortality rates, but it didn't, and it made the rate for maternal morbidity skyrocket. The medical establishment is now backing off internal monitoring and internal catheters. Now the latest technology is geared toward cervical ripening through prostaglandin E2, RU-40, and other forms of chemical management. I talk about this trend: how first they took us from the home and put us in the hospital, and then they developed technology to hold us there. And now that these technologies aren't working, they are moving on to chemical management. To whatever degree possible, the medical establishment looks toward controlling the uterus, and toward controlling the woman around the uterus—that's the way I see it. And I will continue to do all I can to see that public health policies for all women, especially women of color, change.

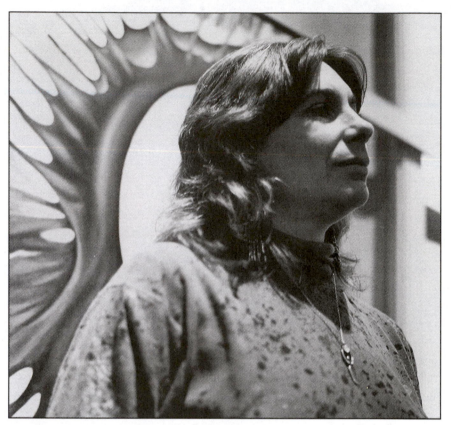

Therese Stallings

Therese Stallings, a direct-entry licensed midwife, is the academic director of the Seattle Midwifery School. She was the first president of MANA, from 1983 to 1986. She has been active on the education committee of MANA and in the Midwives Association of Washington State, the Certification Task Force of the North American Registry of Midwives, and the National Coalition of Midwifery Educators, and the Midwifery Education and Accreditation Council. She lives on Bainbridge Island, a ferry ride from Seattle. One of her current passions is performing with a drumming and singing group and doing women's ritual and movement groups.

Therese Stallings

I decided to be a midwife in a flash. Midwifery is an ancient archetype that comes bubbling out into our brains. I had never met a midwife. I don't know how I even knew the word *midwife*. I had never seen a birth. I had never been pregnant myself and had no association with women's health or midwifery. I was in my early twenties and had been following my free spirit for a few years. I knew it was time to shift and focus my energy, talent, and intelligence and apply myself. It was a summer when I was wrestling with what direction I should take. Then one morning I got up really early and took a walk on the beach, and it just came to me. I don't know from where. At that point, I started putting pieces together. I decided to enroll in nursing school, where I could start getting basic sciences and basic health care. I found out I was pregnant the week I started nursing school. Everything just fell into place—the maternity nursing part of it was very immediate and very relevant and I ate it up.

I think it was 1973 when the inspiration came to me, and it was 1979 before I actually started midwifery training. I worked with dying people for a while. I accompanied a few people on births. Then the Seattle Midwifery School (SMS) opened. I just wasn't the type of person who was going to do midwifery without any training, and there weren't any midwives to apprentice to then. The founding mothers of the Seattle Midwifery School put themselves through the pilot program and then opened it for the first class— for those who were brave and foolish. The school was a really wonderful

experience for me. After graduation I stayed minimally involved. I always had an SMS student in my practice. To me it was bottom line, you always trained a student, and I relied on the student very heavily as birth assistant and for moral support.

Midwifery pointed me in the direction of getting more in touch with the feminine and women's ways. Of course, when I first tackled it, I did it in a left-brain way. I got my education. Then I was very much caught up with proving myself to the boys [meaning the doctors]. That was very important to me, and, oh, the heartache and the frustration that I felt, because of course I was never going to be good enough, and the boys were never going to approve as long as I was a midwife doing homebirth. When I first started my clinic I had it in the basement of a little house that had been renovated into a professional office space. Then we decided to move it into a medical clinic to see if that would make us more legitimate. We were there for about a year and a half until we were pushed out because the doctors didn't want us there when we didn't have malpractice insurance. I really wanted to prove myself to them on their terms. I wanted to show that I was intelligent and competent—all those ways that they measure. Of course, it didn't work. Then I finally came around to having that crisis with myself of realizing how out of touch I was with the feminine and how much, even though I claimed I was doing women's work, I was really doing it in the male model, without even realizing it. My own very personal feelings about myself were not grounded in a feminine center, they were grounded in a masculine judgment, in a masculine evaluation of how much I did.

That's why I say that midwifery work took me through some powerful transformations, for myself personally, and I know obviously for the women that I worked with. One of the things that I stumbled onto was the whole notion of the feminine versus the masculine way of being in the world. The masculine way is to do, to produce, to be out there—action. And the feminine way is to be. I realized that I simply didn't feel good about myself unless I was doing—if I just sat home with a sick kid, with my daughter for the day, I wasn't out there doing something in this way that our culture defines as doing something, so I felt like a nothing, like a zero. What I realized was that the feminine side of me was very underdeveloped. And I thought, Oh my God! Here I am doing this work, supposedly centered around the feminine, but I'm not centered in my own feminine. I am not happy with myself unless I'm doing things, and proving myself in that masculine model. And that was a very important and deeply sobering realization. It set me on a path of coming

to grips with that aspect in myself and trying to work really hard to get comfortable and centered in my beingness. At this point, I finally feel like there is a good balance between my left and my right brain, between my feminine and my masculine. I really get out there and do, but I'm also really good at sitting and just being, and not feeling guilty anymore.

I think if I were going to do midwifery again I would do it differently. One of the things that I've often thought is that I would be more creative with my clients in terms of how I spend time with them. I would do more singing, and more therapeutic touch and visualization. I always did the standard medical things—blood pressure, check weight and measure fundal height [measurement of the uterus's, and hence the baby's, growth], and I would talk and listen. But I was always afraid to just really be truly centered in kind of a more feminine way, without being judged as weird or flaky. I was shy about it. I think I've learned how not to be so driven in that perfectionism, which I think is part of what kept me really busy as a midwife. I wanted to have all those loose ends tied up. There's a certain point where you have to as a midwife. You've got to have that birth kit stocked. You can't show up at a birth and not be organized. You still have to be left-brained. You still have to know how to keep things together.

As a midwife, a feminine part of myself was evoked. A newborn baby hasn't done anything, and yet I love newborn babies. They are probably my favorite part about midwifery—they're just fresh and I would have unconditional love for a newborn baby. This baby hasn't done anything to earn my love, the baby just is, and that love *is* because of that essence, not because of what somebody's done to prove that they are lovable. And then I asked myself, Can I treat myself that way?

Now I feel that I'm learning that I can set limits, and I can say that I'm not going to do, do, do every minute that I'm awake, because that's what makes me feel like I'm a valid good person. I'm going to take some of my days off and I'm just going to sit around and listen to the birds out in my meadow, and listen to music and dance, and sip my cup of tea on my porch, and watch the leaves unfold in the spring.

I went to births for nine years, and I attended three or four hundred births during that time. I started having nightmares the second year I was in training. Total panic dreams—three times a night, year after year after year. They weren't about midwifery; it was just a general anxiety and panic about my security, like losing my wallet or my keys or forgetting my kids somewhere. So at first I didn't relate it to midwifery, but I finally realized the

connection between how my midwifery work aggravated an original wound in me. When this realization came, it was like a lightning bolt. At five in the morning after doing two births one night, without a partner, and without a student, where I had to drive forty miles between the two places, and it was just by the grace of God that I got them both done, without either woman being left in the lurch, it just came to me like, No, Therese, no, you can't keep doing this. I really came to a crisis, and I decided to quit practicing midwifery. My ego was all connected to my role as a midwife because it really feeds the ego, in a way that makes you feel good about yourself. So for years I just didn't want to look at it. But my nervous system simply couldn't handle it. I went to therapy and dealt with some childhood issues that needed to be addressed. My mother was mentally ill when I was growing up, and my panic as a child was that I was responsible for my mother. I had to keep her grounded and safe, and if I didn't do that my survival was at stake—my safety, my security.

I finally realized that every time a woman called me and needed me to ground her in pain, whether she was in labor or she was bleeding and needed me to figure out what to do, it was provoking that primal fear in me. It was reenacting my childhood drama and challenging my fearful child inside. Basically, at my core is a child who didn't feel safe. I can't ever erase that. That's not anything I can undo. I can do what I can to make her strong and safe now, but that child is always going to have that fear and panic in there, so to do midwifery work was constantly to rub salt in that wound. I was in a continuous state of fear and anxiety. I couldn't do it and keep my equilibrium. Even doing the work that I do now, there's that part of me that carries my mother's fear and anxiety.

I don't miss practicing midwifery. I know that I can't do it. I know that I was transformed by the hundreds of births that I attended. I was deepened. I had an understanding of women's wisdom. All that I am in terms of my women-centered spirituality is a result of experiencing birth in that context. I'm really so glad that I did it. I have no regrets. I know that even though I'm not practicing anymore, this will never be taken away from me, that I did get the gift that midwifery has to give.

People were really empathetic and supportive through this transition when I went to the Seattle Midwifery School to be the academic director. I got positive strokes for this, because people felt like that was a wonderful place for me to put my energy and that midwifery wasn't losing me. I do the nitty-gritty of day-to-day operations—making up the class schedule; making

the clinical placements with the students; doing student advising; working on the curriculum to keep it updated; attending faculty meetings, student progress committee meetings, and education council meetings, where we determine our policies; and handling admissions. I also co-teach a course called Midwifery Seminar.

We draw wonderful women to the school, and it's a transformative experience for them. It's very much like what birth does for women. The process of becoming a midwife is just as transformative as having a baby. I don't feel like I'm the one who has everything to teach the students. They all come with rich resources as these wonderful women, so they have a lot to give back. We're the experts in midwifery and that's why they come to the school, but they have all kinds of other things to share. As a staff, we're all really tight. There is a sense of working in a women's supported environment, where you can come to work and feel like you're at home with people and you can share what's going on in your life. You can share how you're feeling, and you can get some slack the days you're not feeling good and give some support the days you are feeling good. Also the preceptors and faculty that we draw in are wonderful women. We've created an incredible place of fifty to sixty people in this community, and I'm the hub of the wheel. I love it. I get a lot out of the rich exchanges between people.

And I like that it's contained to a certain number of hours per week. The fact of the matter is that the job could be full-time but isn't, and even then I wouldn't get everything done. So it's been a very good exercise in letting go of perfectionism and letting go of needing to be right, because I make mistakes all the time, and I have to own them: "Oops, sorry I forgot to tell you that; I just blew it." I have to say that at least once a day, more than once a day, and not feel like I'm a bad person, or guilty.

I do more for midwifery because I'm on the Midwives' Alliance of North America's Education Committee, I'm also on the Interorganizational Work Group (IWG) and on the National Coalition of Midwifery Educators (NCME). This has been a really good time in my life for setting limits on how much am I willing to give to midwifery. Because the first ten years I did midwifery, I just gave it everything. I ate, slept, and drank midwifery. It's such a passion. It has the capacity to really draw that energy out of us, but the fact of the matter is that for me it just burned me up. My lesson now was how can I do this work, and have a life and have energy for other things too.

I think a basic issue why American women have such a hard time giving birth is because they are not in their bodies. I can see that because I'm not

doing births now, I'm moving in the direction of midwifing women into their bodies. It's a preliminary step to preparing them for birth. I use African rhythms and drums because they are so powerful—they move you if you can just relax and really be moved. I'm trying to facilitate that process. It's not really teaching specific dance steps as much as how to let go of self-consciousness and be fully incarnate in your body, and then just let the music move you in a way that just creates this great joy and ecstacy. That's the trick of it; to get that kind of participation and to inspire people that, yes, even though you are a white honkey, you too can move, and can be fully, entirely in your body. This is where my passion is right now, and I can see that women in America aren't ready for midwives yet. There are some missing pieces—they're not connected to their bodies, so of course they don't trust midwives to take care of them in a homebirth. So we can start with acknowledging that and try to educate women through their brains, but it's much deeper than that, it's cellular. You can talk all you want to the head and it doesn't connect, and so doing movement and education will hopefully be the thing that will help shift that. It certainly has been for me.

I have been really touched and changed by the women I've met in my organizational work for midwives in the Midwives' Alliance of North America. I had been in student body politics in high school and have always been a kind of an organizational person. I had skills from being involved in starting a food co-op, and sitting on boards [of directors], but my first inspiration to get involved in midwifery organization was Sister Angela [Murdaugh]. She was like her name, "the angel." She touched my heart and said, "This is really important for midwifery. Midwives need an organization that is going to address some of the concerns and move midwifery forward. I've called you people here, because you're the key people as near as I can identify, to get this to happen." Of course I just said, "All right, Sister Angela. I've got it. I've got it."

I was really very moved by her and so full of zeal that I picked up the ball and ran with it. I became the first MANA president and just devoted my life to it—and that's part of why I burned out, as I was running a pretty busy practice at the time as well. It really changed me to interface with midwives from all over the country. I think lay midwives came to midwifery in such an inspired way.

And now, if there is anything that I'm good at, it's group process, because of years of meetings with MANA. I had years of listening to people and hammering out a course of action based on varying viewpoints. I've learned

an enormous amount—like how to be able to listen to everybody and be able to understand everybody's position, really understand it, and empathize with it, even though it's not mine. We all have a tendency to want to put people into categories, because it's easier to deal with them that way, but it's not fair, and assumptions are made that aren't correct. I started to gain an ability to just lay down my own perspective and truly hear and understand how somebody else came to something in a totally different way than I would have done it.

I feel like midwives in America right now are keeping something alive for the women of America that the culture is not keeping alive and honoring. It's really a struggle for all of us to keep it alive. Are we like a flickering flame, like a pilot light that at some point somebody's going to turn on the gas, and we're going to ignite? Or is it just this little flickering flame that we're struggling so hard just to keep it from getting blown out? I think my current belief is that we're just at the point where I don't think it's going to catch, direct-entry midwifery in particular. I think nurse-midwives are catching, though not in the form that we think (and even a lot of the nurse-midwives think) is ideal midwifery. They don't like working in those big group practices, where they are just worked like dogs and they don't have continuity of care, and they don't get all that satisfaction either. But that's the kind of midwifery the world wants. The kind of midwifery that we do, that wonderful personal continuity of care, honoring the natural process, that is sitting by women's bedsides, whether it be for two days or what . . . that is not catching on, but thank God we're keeping it alive.

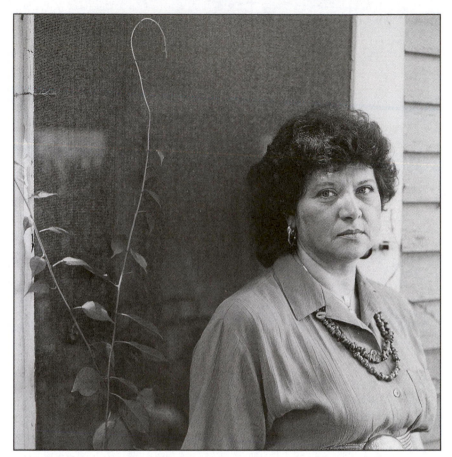

Fran Ventre

Fran Ventre first became a midwife in the 1970s after being certified as a childbirth educator by the American Society for Psychoprophylaxis in Obstetrics in 1972. She began attending homebirths in her community and was the first modern-day lay midwife to be licensed in the state of Maryland, challenging an old law that was still on the books. She became a nurse-midwife in 1978 after attending Georgetown University, and in 1991 received a master's in public health from Boston University. Fran was responsible for developing and starting the first licensed birth center in Massachusetts in collaboration with Beverly Hospital in 1980. She was the director for four years of this freestanding birth center, which is still in operation. She has since worked in a number of nurse-midwifery practices in the Boston area and is currently a nurse-midwife with Harvard Community Health Plan attending births at Brigham and Women's Hospital.

Fran has been active in both of the national midwifery organizations. She was one of the founding mothers of and the first regional representative of New England to MANA, from 1982 to 1985, and has been the chair of the Boston area chapter of the ACNM. She envisions a "Bridge Club" in MANA and ACNM for midwives who have worked both as independent and nurse-midwives. Her articles on lay midwifery and homebirth were some of the first published in the *Journal of Nurse-Midwifery, Birth and the Family Journal,* and *Compulsory Hospitalization: Freedom of Choice in Childbirth?* She was also the co-founder of HOME (home-oriented maternity experience) in 1973 and edited their newsletter for six years.

Fran Ventre

I have a vision of a film that I want to make to really give people an idea of what birth is about. In this vision there is music, a whole orchestra, people's faces when they are running marathons or lifting weights with the noise they are making and their intense emotions. I would juxtapose various times of labor with all these visions and emotions. Because, what I see when women have early, or what they call Braxton-Hicks false labor [intermittent contractions that sometimes precede labor contractions]—I hate those terms—is like an orchestra tuning up. When an orchestra tunes up, each instrument plays randomly and it sounds like noise—but this is a necessary and creative noise. The musicians are all tuning their instruments. And it isn't until the instruments are tuned that the conductor raises the baton and the orchestra plays together in concert and harmony the way the muscles do when labor starts in earnest. And it's also like an athlete warming up before a marathon. Labor transition is like running Heartbreak Hill of the Boston Marathon— the pain and sweat that the runners suffer is intense, and yet there is so much glory with that. My son ran the Boston Marathon for the first time a few years ago, and he said it was so hard and that he just wanted to throw up at one point, and I thought, Wow, that sounds like labor. When I stood at the finish line waiting for him and looked at the faces of everyone coming in I thought there was an aura around every one of those runners. They were exhausted, but their faces were radiant with exhilaration. It's the same thing with birth, looking at a new mother's face.

Sometimes in hospitals where there are many epidurals [regional anesthesia used to deaden the sensation of contractions during labor or for surgery], the whole labor area is quiet. So if you don't order an epidural and the woman is making noise, the nurse will say to the midwife, "She's really in pain. She's making a lot of noise!" My answer to that is, "Well, wouldn't it be weird if you went to an amusement park and you didn't hear any noise at the roller coaster ride? Noise is okay." And it's okay to have pain, to sweat, to make noise. Yet in labor, people say that unless the laboring mother is absolutely stoic, then she should have drugs or an epidural. I have been accused of withholding drugs, of making women suffer, but I come from a unique background from which I have witnessed women's empowerment by their birth experiences.

At the birth center where I used to work, there was such a range of people. Some didn't really know what they were in for or what the philosophy was. But by experiencing the natural process they got to understand how birth can empower them.

At a birth center or homebirth, no drugs are available for them, and it is actually easier to resist interference than for those who are in the hospital. We used to call it the "candy-on-the-shelf" theory, because when you go to the hospital, it's like when you take your kid into the candy store and then say, "No, you can't eat the candy. You've got to have carrots and celery and rice crackers." I believe that there shouldn't be any drugs available at a birth center, because once you get into the drugs, you would need a fetal monitor to see how the drugs are affecting the baby's well-being and heart rate. Instead, at a homebirth or birth center, there are other options like warm baths—and the partners or support people at the birth are freer to play a more active role. People who didn't initially even know or understand what they were going to get at the birth center and who came because it was an "in" thing to do, came out saying, "Wow, I didn't know that I could do that!" And that is no small thing that a parent comes away from a birth saying, "I can do this." It is a very empowering feeling. Some people will say, "Oh, you people just want your experience for the experience." Well, of course—why do people climb Mount Everest or run the marathon? And it is that power that can carry them through the adjustments to parenting.

I began to get involved in midwifery in the 1970s, which was kind of a utopian time, a Camelot era for midwifery. Some people when they talk about the seventies and the whole flower child era put it down. But I say, no that was a special time when people who were choosing homebirths did it

because of a very strong commitment to birth, and to me as a midwife it affected the way that I was serving them. Unfortunately, some aspects of that lifestyle got out of hand with drugs, but the concept of communes was wonderful. There was such a good spirit there—I used to love attending their births.

I was the middle-class, Chevy Chase housewife going off to the communes, and different religious groups were always trying to recruit me to the fold. People also understood that if they wanted me at their births that there would be times when I would have to bring my kids. And my kids knew that when my husband was out of town, they would be awakened in the middle of the night and they would have to come with me. Even if my husband was in town, I didn't want to call him home from work because at the time I wasn't making any money and since he didn't like cooking back then, he often took them out to dinner. He said it was costing us a fortune my being a midwife. He was very supportive of my midwife activities, but he was also concerned about the legalities and the chance that I could be sued. I assured him that it would never happen—but it was a different group of people then, with a different mindset. And I often wonder now, where have all the "flowers" gone?

I also developed a strong support system—I lived in a neighborhood where my friends helped me. When I was not at a birth, I took care of everyone else's kids so that their mothers owed me so much child care time that if I had to impose on them, they'd be grateful that they could finally pay me back. I did it that way so I wouldn't feel guilty when I took off and I would have to call friends to pick up my three kids after school. Now that my kids are adults they look back and understand and say that they are proud of what I did. They knew of my strong commitment to midwifery, and I tried hard not to let them feel that I neglected them, and tried to work things out for them. I would never make commitments to them that I couldn't keep. They knew that planned activities were contingent upon no one being in labor. And when I had HOME meetings and La Leche League [a breastfeeding support, referral, and information group] groups at my house, they were always around and included. They'd sometimes complain and say, "You and your hippie friends." But today they say, "Gee, Mom. Thanks for breastfeeding us for so long, because we really got very healthy," and they fondly remember all those people and babies coming to the house. Today they've all become health conscious and appreciate their healthy beginnings.

I was deeply committed to my family, so it was a juggling act. There

were times when I would be up for forty-eight hours straight and then come back on a Sunday morning when we had our ritual Sunday brunch. My husband and kids were cooking and I wouldn't go to sleep, as exhausted as I was—I would come in and cook with them and sit down and have the brunch. When they went off to their own activities, then I would go to sleep; otherwise I would often put it off. They came through it fine—I think they are terrific young people. As much as I've done as a midwife, which I'm pretty proud of, I feel proudest that my kids turned out so well. So midwifery didn't hurt them—but you have to do more, especially when you go to homebirths or birth center births—as midwifery is not a job but a part of your life. I was also fortunate to have a supportive husband who encouraged me and also had a strong commitment to family. When you attend births in a hospital it doesn't often require as much devotion, and you don't have that kind of intense relationship with the women. Often there is a team of midwives.

The birth center that I started in 1980 with another CNM was like my baby. It was a place where women could have a dignified birth experience. We wanted the birth center to be beautiful and impeccably clean so that it showed the respect we had for the environment of birth. I sewed window shades that matched the wallpaper. I remember arguing with one of the hospital administrators about the curtains. He wanted me to pick out special fireproof materials because to him the birth center was an institution. But the fabrics were so ugly! And I said, "You don't understand—we need to have beautiful fabrics and warm colors. It affects how you feel. Nice fabrics can be treated so that they are fireproof." And he said, "Fran, you're getting carried away with this; you'd think it was your own home you were decorating!" And I said, "That's it. You've got it."

The women got involved then. They made bedspreads, and one woman took our logo and embroidered it with a heart that had the name of her child with the weight and date of birth. So when the next baby was born we put up another similar heart, and it became a tradition. And when the kids went there, they would look for their birth heart. A birth center belongs to the community—people should feel they can come in at any time and put a piece of themselves there, and they would be inspired, want to keep it beautiful.

We never said at the birth center, "Well, it's housekeeping's job to clean up." We wanted it to always look wonderful and aesthetically pleasing. We didn't care if we were midwives, we got down and scrubbed to maintain it. Then it becomes a respected place, it becomes hallowed and the community respects it because they know this is a space that takes care of them. By mak-

ing it a beautiful space you are telling the people who are coming there what you think of them. And I don't mean you have to buy expensive furnishings—we got some of the best things at thrift shops. What I mean is showing your love and caring through making it beautiful.

When I left the birth center I felt I had lost a child. I've done and left other things, but that was so deep in my soul. It was a real death for me. Separating from the other midwives who worked there was like a divorce. So it took a long time to heal from that. I left because of philosophical changes in clinical practice that were threatening to happen. I felt that many changes being imposed would compromise the ideals of the birth center and impose more restrictions—making the birth center more an adaptation of the hospital than a homelike environment. These new protocols were being imposed by new OBs joining the consulting OBs, and I felt like I would be betraying the families.

At that point I took nine months off, and I thought maybe I didn't want to be a midwife anymore. I thought about doing something else or returning to being a schoolteacher. I went on a trip to Puerto Rico with my husband, and he had to go off on business, so I rented a car and went exploring on my own. Interestingly, I met women in out-of-the-way places, and invariably, without even knowing me, these women would get to telling me about their life and their experiences in childbearing. And I didn't always let it be known that I was a midwife. I wanted people to acknowledge me for myself—not always "Fran-the-midwife," because for a good part of my adult life I was known primarily as a midwife and I was experiencing an "identity crisis." I was in search of my true identity. And what I discovered in that time alone, driving through the winding mountain roads in Puerto Rico, was that midwifery was merely the vehicle or vessel for me, through which I can express that identity. And when that revelation came to me, I said, "OK, that's who I am. I am a midwife." And that's when I came back to midwifery and what I have chosen. Some people express themselves through their music, some through their writing, or whatever they do best. For me, being a midwife defines who I am and what I believe in. It is my calling.

Presently I work as a midwife in a hospital and I've learned that birth experiences are very different in a place like a tertiary-care center [where care is given for high-risk patients] in contrast to a homebirth or at a birth center. But there was a time when I used to be very smug in that sense and felt that you were really not a midwife unless you were doing homebirths. But now, having worked in different environments, I really believe you can be a mid-

wife anywhere—and a lot of that is determined by the women and what their expectations are and your own commitment to the women. I can just try to do the best I can to be with women when they have their babies, wherever it is. Homebirths and birth centers are admittedly something very special, and I would want my children to have that kind of experience for their births. But we can try to duplicate that philosophy and keep that vision as much as possible in the hospital. And as long as women choose to go to hospitals for birth, I would hope that there will be midwives for them.

One of the positive things about working as a midwife in the hospital is that nurses and the other staff get to see normal midwifery births now. They used to only see midwives and homebirth couples in a crisis situation, when there was a problem with a laboring woman or baby that needed to be transferred in. Once I had a situation where a nurse asked, "Fran, could you be on standby? The doctor is not here and this woman is a multip [had one baby already], and she had an urge to push." So I ran in her room, and I realized that she's not fully dilated and I said, "Oh, she's not fully dilated. I'm sure the doctor will be here in time."

And I just knelt at the foot of her bed and locked eyes with her and I don't know why but I just bonded to this woman unbelievably, instantaneously. I felt like I'd known her always. I said "Your doctor will be here soon . . ."

And she said, "I hope you won't leave; I love looking at your face." My face . . . in the middle of the night! Then she started pushing and her doctor came in and she said to me, "No, don't take your hands off . . . I want you here."

She had a perfect birth, and her doctor was just standing there. I had a sinking feeling like I might get into big trouble. So I joked with him afterward to keep it light and said, "You know, I didn't really know what to do. I felt like she wanted me to stay. I felt like Sally Fields when she accepted her Academy Award: 'You like me, You really like me.' I hope you weren't offended." Fortunately, he had a sense of humor.

But he saw all of this "touchy-feely" stuff. Unfortunately, this aspect of birth isn't always acknowledged as important. I see it even with some new midwives, nurse-midwives who come from a high-risk background and whose midwifery education often reinforces the scientific approach. They think I'm sometimes too laid back, that I don't *do* enough. But with time and experience I would hope that they learn to mellow and trust birth. In some ways the midwifery that is becoming more accepted in this country is becom-

ing more medical. Maybe there's a certain need to do that in this day and age. It is a dilemma for all midwives today—the balance between doing something or just trusting the natural process. We need the education and the credentials but we need to hold on to and reinforce what MANA represents, and that's the soul or spirit of midwifery.

The hardest part of being a midwife is the ongoing political struggle. Sometimes you get so tired of it, weary of having to prove yourself, and tired of saying, "We belong here. We have a right to be midwives." One of the older midwives calls us "the walking wounded of midwifery." We all get wounded at one time or another. I don't think there's any midwife who hasn't been deeply wounded in the continual political struggle. And we are so beholden to the medical establishment in order even to be allowed to practice. That's the hard part—that they have so much say over how we can practice or where we can practice. If I wanted to start a birth center here now I could open one right up if I were a doctor. But if I started a private midwifery service and have a backup doctor and something happened [had to relocate, or was pressured by colleagues or hospital] to that person, my whole business would go down the tubes. I don't know when that will change. I think that when you are practicing outside of the system you can be a little more independent, and I know some nurse-midwives object to the term *independent midwife* for *lay midwife*. However there are some very real negative aspects of being outside of the system that are very hard to deal with—you're very isolated and very vulnerable. I know—I've lived it.

When I left the birth center I was accused of being too radical and not willing to compromise, and I felt like what Kitty Ernst [a CNM who has been active in the promotion of birth centers and in community-based nurse-midwifery education] once described about midwives at once part of the system and yet outside of it. We are in a rowboat drifting off and we have one foot in the rowboat and one on land. We don't know whether to jump ashore or to go in the rowboat. We get split apart, pulled in both directions.

Now with the two midwifery organizations, MANA and ACNM, I often don't know to which group I really belong. I'm like the leprechaun who sang the song in *Finian's Rainbow*, "When I'm not near the girl I love, I love the girl I'm near." When I was with MANA midwives and heard nurse-midwives being put down or negative things, I'd get very defensive. And then when I'd be with the other group, as a member of the ACNM and heard the direct-entry or lay midwife be put down, I'd get very defensive. I was always feeling that I was defending the other and that it was hard to be in

that position. It's schizophrenic, but right now I can see the appropriateness of MANA representing the interests and philosophy of the direct-entry midwives.

I was always very impressed with the creative way that the MANA board worked. In the past, we had some terrible meetings. One time when I was on the MANA board I was arguing with another midwife during a board meeting—I was so mad at her I hated her. But that night we had a party and she started disco dancing and I danced with her. We all danced and the rancor of the meeting dissipated. How could you continue to hate someone when you were having so much fun dancing with her? The next day at the board meeting, I had a totally different feeling about her. I still disagreed with her opinions, but I didn't feel that personal animosity. I could now be more open to her perspective. It was like I could acknowledge her and really enjoy who she was. MANA knows how to incorporate *play*—which helps with grounding us to the real purpose of keeping the soul of midwifery alive.

At another MANA board meeting when I was no longer on the board, I offered to be the "mother" and cook and take care of the midwife board members. This meeting was at one of the midwive's houses to save money, and I wanted to nurture and take care of them while they did the business of MANA. I think that this is women's way of taking care of business. We are accustomed to accomplishing great feats and doing creative things at our dining room tables. I remember as a young mother when I was involved in La Leche League and I never had an office. People always came to my house, and the most constructive ideas and things were accomplished by just talking a lot. Sometimes I'm accused of not getting right to the point, and to me it's okay if we ramble on, back and forth, interrupting each other, because this is how our ideas flow.

On the other hand, the ACNM, which represents me as a nurse-midwife, has done much with education and has become an important professional business organization which is very effective in lobbying and legislating for us locally and nationally to make midwifery legitimate. As an organization it is the "big sister." But the ACNM is also evolving and beginning to recognize that midwifery is a profession separate from nursing. The two organizations are really like the two arms of women, and ultimately someday I would like to see the two arms come together and embrace the body of midwifery.

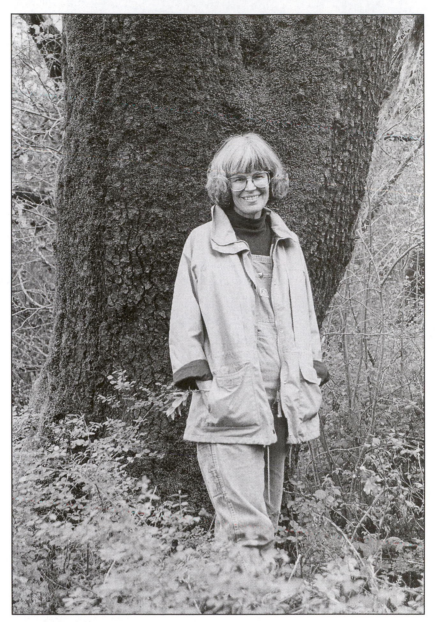

Candace Whitridge

Candace Whitridge was in the first class of nurse-midwives to graduate from the University of California—San Francisco, in 1978. She is a family nurse practitioner as well as a CNM. She has worked in many health and human service organizations, focusing on children's and women's rights and abuse prevention, and has been the first vice-president of MANA. She runs an organic family farm in northern California, has been the president of the Trinity County Organic Growers Association, and edits a monthly farming newsletter. As a midwife and ecofeminist, Candace travels internationally to speak on the art of positive prenatal care and ecological reflections on birth and feminism. Candace is a student of Buddhism.

Candace Whitridge

Anyone who farms or gardens knows that it is a myth that farmers grow food and midwives deliver babies. I realized early on that the women that I used to attend were delivering their own babies and that I was really their assistant. It's the woman who is growing the baby, and so my whole focus was on her. I'm not doing anything any differently farming than I did as a midwife. As a farmer my focus is on the earth, so through covercropping, composting, respect for the soil, building up the soil, keeping it fertile, keeping it healthy—then that healthy soil is going to grow a plant. It's not like I don't watch to see if the plants are growing, but I don't in any way think that I'm growing that food. I don't focus on the plant separate from the earth.

When you farm, the farther away you get from the earth, you get really out of touch. It doesn't mean that you can't grow massive amounts of food, harvest it all, ship it all out, and be serving the planet, but your understanding of the process starts deteriorating the farther away that you get. For me, if I could do it, I would do everything with my hands. I would reach down deep and till with my hands. I would weed with my hands. I use my fingers, I don't put gloves on. When I do that, it feels like I have an understanding that's beyond vocabulary of what's going on. I look at every single plant. I know when the earth needs water and doesn't need water. There is an energy in the food.

And there is energy in women and babies, and that gets lost when you are giving them little perfunctory prenatal visits that are all only measure-

ments or monitoring. Some people don't even feel the woman's belly any-more. They're just doing serial ultrasounds, measuring the bones to see if they equal the number of weeks that's on her chart. They do all this almost like the woman is a vehicle for the baby. The woman should eat well because she's the mainline for the food for the baby. They know the position, because they see it on this little picture. No matter that they are blasting this kid with sound waves. Everybody hooked up. It's expedient to just look in with all these monitors. That's what's happening with farming. I hate to sit in judg-ment of things, but it worries me. I think that when you look at just the evolution of life, that we're on our way out when we do this.

I think when you take care of a woman, and as you're measuring her the praise really goes, "You can see how well you're caring for yourself. Look how your child is thriving." There is language that should be present all the time through prenatal visits. To affirm her work, that she knows what she's doing, and when things are not proper, it's just like fine-tuning our lives.

I teach classes on prenatal care, because I think there is a whole language around what we do. Even around how we feel the baby or how we check a blood pressure. I think we can get so caught up in all the little routines that we forget that women have all their pores open during preg-nancy. All we need to do is just to continue to saturate them with good feelings and images so that they float out of your office in a serene state.

I have learned my whole philosophy of prenatal care through the women I have taken care of. They've been amazing teachers when I spend a lot of time with them. As they begin to share their lives and their thoughts and things, I develop a deeper understanding of what the use of language does to women, the subtleties of certain words, the subtleties of the way you do exams, the kinds of things that help a woman sort of peel off these little layers of themselves, an encrusted sort of mud that comes from us through the things that we hear in society. To somehow peel this stuff away so that the knowledge that they forgot, they remember. Very few women have any knowledge that the resources really are present in them. We truly believe that something outside of us, above us, apart from us is where the wisdom really lies. It was a focus for me to somehow have the little jewel in them begin to materialize for themselves. Who they are, not how I wanted to see any of them. I began to look at all those things that would just nurture them and I'd fuss and cluck and make women feel incredible during their pregnancies. I thought the more powerful a woman began to feel that it would have a total

impact on the birth. And as midwives we were really guides for them, and prenatal care was really our opportunity to affirm *their* work.

You know when you put two people in a relationship there's this funny little dance you do when you first meet until you shift into something that's a rhythm. Almost inevitably, if you're looking at a health care person and a client, the client will make a shift, because they are really going to try to please you, so they accommodate to you. They accommodate to you in ways that are so subtle that they don't even realize that they are doing it.

I think it is a big difference if we just immediately go to them. Some of this is even in the way we use our voice, or in posturing, or our presence. I think that it subtly says to the woman that they've met someone who is already appreciating who they are. I don't know how to put this in words. Women don't have to start changing themselves. They don't have to be reserved if they're not or pretend to be talkative if they're not, so that they can fit this dance with you. Then they reveal to you things about themselves and about their family that really allows for you to care for them better. The relationship was one of those things that gently and slowly evolves and gets deep. The rhythm was not broken up.

Moving into the woman's labor and birth was just kind of a continuation of the relationship we started in prenatal care. It just seemed smooth to me. For me the presence I had at the birth would be much of my knowledge of who they were, and my respect for them. So my presence at each birth would be as different with each woman as it was during prenatal care. For some people, I was actually present in another room or quietly sitting in a corner, and I did nothing other than to listen to the baby's pleasure and displeasure at the journey. But it required nothing, no words, no exams, nothing.

For some women I think that much of our job is really being the anchor for them, so that they can get way out there and look over to see that you are smiling and giving them a nod and a little "mmmm" that they are fine. For other people there needs to be a little more active participation.

It's planting things that you want to be part of their memory of birth. What you want them to remember are all those positive things. Because women are so open at birth, you have to be really careful with the language that people use. During the most powerful time of opening, that stuff will all go in there. It fuels their efforts at the time, but that also is the stuff that finds its home in there.

Pregnancy and birth are an imaginative time. It's just imagining how you would be at a birth, or imagining yourself as a mother. You're sort of

tickling with your potential, that part of your womanhood. It's not so real, and with birth it starts becoming real, and then parenthood is just there.

People can start getting confused about what they should do in [parenting] situations. They think that there is going to be some formula that is going to tell them what to do when their baby cries and doesn't stop. And what do they do with sleep deprivation, and how do they make their relationship work with their partner again now that there's a child and no time for sex? These are hard-core realities that are affecting them now day-to-day. I think that our role is to give them some guidance through the maze of all this, mostly through story-telling, and assuring them that a sense of humor through this entire process is just so important.

For me a lot of prenatal care was the talks that you had. The things where you both came away different after every visit, because you begin to rise above mediocrity, rise above those mundane things of life. Your spirit could sort of take flight as women talking together. You reach into yourself on things that sort of just come forth, that you don't actually tap into otherwise. We get so busy in our lives—it's hard for us. Maybe we might read an inspiring book, or you catch a moment with a friend. It's part of a spiritual life of women. I felt for me that a lot of the prenatal care for women was in fact these opportunities. Women used to just long for their prenatal visits, because it's hard to have that sort of talk when your lives are busy, and to be in a place where the door would be closed and she knew that there was like a little hour of sanctuary time.

I had a little woman's health care center called the Mountain Clinic. It was pretty funky, relaxed—it was just a home; it wasn't like an office. It was not high volume. All the families would be in there all the time. It was actually kind of a community hangout. They were very involved in all the care, and with all the kids running around and stuff—it was like life is, and it should be for women.

For me, in a community like this, I just continue to grow up with all these women. What an incredible thing for these kids—to be living somewhere where they are absolutely aware at this age of having been born. Their mothers gave them birth, and there was a woman in their community who assisted their mother, whom they have a relationship with. At the school, I'm really all the time having kids coming around, and they know me through this relationship. I was there at their birth, and they tell people that. They talk about it. Most of us have no idea to even think about our own births. They tell people about their own births. They know that they were born, and that it

was happy. Their attitudes about this are really very positive. Most of these people have photographs and they have pictures in books, and for many of these children it's a ritual for them on their birthdays to go back and hear the story of their birth. It's like a fairy tale recounted over and over again.

So for me the postpartum care goes on and on and on. It's just the village relationships that happen—there's a rhythm that continues. It's not these segmented things. It's just meeting people and beginning to develop a bond of respect with them. One that is going to endure so that you don't have to hurry up and have a deep, meaningful relationship fast. I'm not so good at these flash-in-the-pan things. I like the ones that just evolve deeper. It's like the oak. It grows a little slowly, but the roots go real deep. It's going to take a lot to knock this down. That's how we are here as friends. We've all, all these people here, we've all known each other for a long time by and large. That's the context in which I wish to be a midwife. I wouldn't do well at a tertiary-care center [where care is given for high-risk patients] because for me, I really want the relationships with people. I want to be just a quiet, gentle presence. I want to be a part of their lives in that way, but not in any dramatic way, not making it more significant than it is.

There's an African folktale about birth. It's like being on a really narrow log on a very shallow, rapidly moving river. The woman is standing on the log, and she's going to get from one side of the shore to the other side. All the people in the village and all her loved ones can walk alongside this log. They can tell her how to keep her balance, and if the woman falls off, they can say, "Don't worry, you're not drowning. This is shallow water. Stand up. See, it's not over your head. Get back on the log." They help her get on the log. They can do all these things. They can tell her how far the shore is, "Looks good. Getting closer. Whoops, you fell off. Well, back on the log. Okay, you need a little food. Rest here." The log gets caught up on a stone, sways a little bit, "It's okay." They can do all those things, but they cannot get on the log. It's a one-person log. Only one person can get on this log.

There is a blessing ceremony that occurs when you are feeling a woman's pelvis. For me I always make kind of a big deal out of it. I say, "Here I am. Now I am feeling the womb. I'm just going to have a little feel of the passage [where the baby will pass through] here of where your bones are and everything." It's like a ceremony, and you can see people waiting for this. They need the blessing.

I take this cloth pelvis. I don't use those bony things. I use those pretend things, so you can show them how flexible it is, to create this whole

imagery of vast space. Then I go, "Whoa, oh right." I say, "Honey child, you were built to have a baby. This is great," and they go, "Ohhh right." It is literally the blessing. Depending on where you live, you can use different imagery. [Because I live in a logging area] I say, "You could drive a truck through this pelvis." "Really?" Sigh.

It's a real important first seed to plant, so when labor starts toughening up, they know that they've just got to work a little harder, dig a little deeper. If someone has planted any shadow of a doubt in them from the beginning, then they're going to go, "Oh, they're right, huh? I'm too small? Something wrong here? I'm not built right. There's something wrong? Maybe this baby can't get out. Is the baby stuck?" You can only imagine the pictures that are starting to go through their heads of their baby battering up against bones that are too small or too tight or too something. What they'll do is that they'll protect that baby and they won't open up any more. You know how many cesarean sections have been done because somebody planted a bad seed in a lady from the beginning? Don't ever place a shadow of a doubt in a woman that she can't do something. You let her just rip into it. Don't have them hold back. You don't have an orgasm if you hold back. You don't experience birth if you hold back.

I have stopped trying to intellectually think about where my life will go with midwifery. What I have discovered and why I have stopped trying to think about it is that I have a deep faith in the universe. It gets deeper every day. I have really been lucky. If I were to die ten minutes from now, I am not holding on to any "I wish I would have's." I believe in reincarnation. I think that whatever I did in my last lifetime was the prelude to my work now. Whatever my work is now and whatever comes to me, whether it be gifts or extreme challenges, I believe that this is all part of my life here. I no longer push or try to determine my way anymore. I have this little tickle in my head all the time that I am going to be catching babies again. Midwifery is so in me. I think it has been in me a long time. I believe that I am going to reap what I sow. That's where choice lies in my life.

I remember almost three years ago my ex-husband (and the father of my daughter) was killed horribly. Before then, I thought I had something that explained why I'm here. Whatever I had, it didn't hold up for one second after his death. I went, "Holy fuck. I don't know what I believe in. I have no idea about death. I don't even know why I'm alive. I don't know anything."

I went into the most profound darkness. It was like I had toxic waste in me that had to come out. I was aware that I was being almost absorbed by

demons just rushing through me. It was extraordinary. I would look at someone and all I could see was what I didn't like about them. Everything that was
in my mind was evil. I finally just had to say, "I've just got to ride this out. I
don't know what is happening to me." Then I had profound dreams of Jim.
He came to me, and I literally think his spirit came to me. I saw him sur-
rounded by light, walking like he was Jesus. I knew he was fine. Then I felt
darkness, literally, it was incredible, just like chunks came off of me and things
started to happen. All of a sudden stuff started to open up to me. It didn't
turn me into some zealot. It was quiet, but I just said, "Oh, God, thank you."
I knew that he was out there passing on something. I don't think that I'm like
some missionary person, but it was like life started. Nothing I articulate.
That's why I no longer try to make anything happen in my life. I finally,
finally surrendered to this. It took death to get life. It takes death to have
birth. It takes death every day. You know what I do all day long? I try. Every
day I rise up and I think about getting hit on a motorcycle by a water truck
ten minutes from now. I contemplate impermanence all day long. I still feel
that even though I'm not catching babies, there's something happening to
me right now that if I'm to go back and catch babies I'm going to be serving
women better than I have before, because of needing to somehow become
wiser. Wisdom comes through the other facets of our lives—it's all just this
continuum. But I think there's something important happening to me right
now. I think I had to go through death and explosive spiritual change and
awareness of things. I want to work hard and be paced cyclically with the
rhythm of the farm and of the community here.

I think there are midwives out there whose lives are screaming at them
to stop practicing right now. They need to put things on hold for a while,
especially when it is so discordant in their families. We hold in our midwifery
practice this ideal of integration of family and love and birth, and yet it's a
paradox when our lives are in shambles around us. I have met some midwives
who I know are clinging to their midwifery because they think it is feeding
them in some way that sustains them. And I think to myself, "You need to let
go of this right now." Sometimes what happens is that they're becoming the
indispensable midwife. Which we have to be very careful that we don't do. As
midwives, we're notorious for substituting as the external factor that women
are dependent on. If you in fact have got people so strongly doing birth
themselves, and you have truly become this little assistant for them, if people
can't even remember who was there at their birth, then I think you have done
a pretty good job.

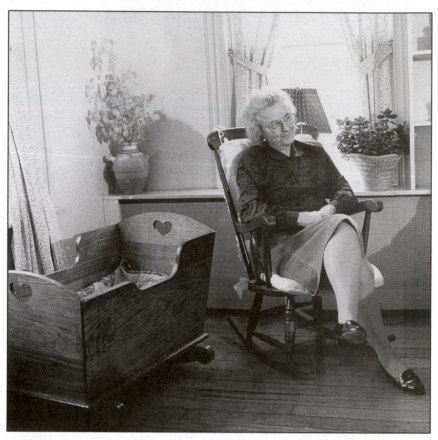

Edie Wonnell

Edie Wonnell is the founder and director of the Birth Center of Delaware, a freestanding birth center that provides well-woman care; childbirth classes (including ones for grandparents); and care during the prenatal, delivery, and postpartum periods. In 1976, she received the Delaware Nurse of the Year Award for her outstanding contribution toward improving the health of mothers and babies. She has been a midwife since 1955 and has attended births at home, in birth centers, and in hospitals. She has been a midwifery instructor in many programs and was on the board of directors of the National Association of Childbearing Centers from 1985 to 1987, which set standards for birth centers to get national accreditation.

Edie Wonnell

I've been a nurse-midwife for thirty-five years, and I was the first childbirth educator to come to the Philadelphia area. The birth center movement was just beginning in the mid seventies when I set up the nurse-midwifery service at the Bryn Mawr Birth Center. I soon began to notice that about 20 percent of our clientele were from Delaware. One very snowy night, I get a telephone call from somebody in Delaware ten minutes away from me who was in labor. We both had to risk our lives traveling an hour in a snowstorm to get to a place where she could have her birth. And I thought, You know, this is absolutely crazy, and so I went about trying to establish a birth center here in Delaware.

Well, this is a terribly conservative state. I had to go through the whole process of getting a certificate of need, developing the document, going before public hearings and against a medical society that was very much opposed to the concept. Fortunately, the committee set up to review had a few key people on it who, in the end, were very influential. I presented the concept and economics, the safety and so forth, and of course the president of the Board of Medicine got up and spoke about how this system would be like going back to medieval times—we would have blood running down the street, the whole scenario. A nurse was there who had read [Mary Breckinridge's] *Wide Neighborhoods* (1981), a book about midwifery, and she stood up and said, "We have a record of nurse-midwives' contribution and the safety of it, even for women in the rural mountain areas of Appalachia." And a

physician who was part of the Veterans' Administration stood up and said, "If we can airlift wounded men out of battlefields, why can't we transfer women half a block?" Well, I could just feel the whole committee at that point say, "Why not?" and it passed.

For the first year we were open I could just visualize the whole medical society sitting on the stoop out front waiting for the first mistake so that they could close us down. And here we are, ten years later, with a perfect safety record, and at this point, I think we have a reputation in the community for delivering excellent care. What I've learned is that it is so important to have people planted in your community who have the vision to see that there are different ways of accomplishing care. Right now we are in a very crucial time in the United States, and we have got to come up with more imaginative ways of providing health care services in all aspects, not only in maternity care.

It's interesting to note that many of the nurses who work for me are nurses who work on labor and delivery or in intensive-care nurseries; they enjoy midwifery because it helps them keep a mental balance, because they never see the normal in the hospital. It brings them back to the reality of what birth should be about. I think the major difference in philosophy between a midwife and a doctor is that the midwife sees birth as a normal, healthy function and the doctor sees it as an emergency about to happen. And that's why I want to see the birth center remain open so that we can demonstrate our belief in practice, not only to the community, but also to the professionals. We're coming out with just as good statistics as they are: we run anywhere between 2 percent and 5 percent cesarean rate.

Out-of-hospital birthing makes you the mother of invention, and I would love to see every nurse-midwife in the country get out of exclusive hospital work so she doesn't lose touch with what I call "real midwifery." Of course, it's nice to have all the technology, but we must not lose faith in our hands and in our heads, and so I think flowing between the two is good.

I would say the main interest in my establishing the birth center here was, number one, to provide a place for nurse-midwives to practice, and secondly, to provide the alternative for patients who do not want to get into the high-tech environment and who believe very strongly that birth is a biological process which we are all prepared for. Although only 15 percent of birthing women need the high-tech equipment, the hospitals are completely geared toward that small minority. That is not to say that hospitals are not important; I believe that the key to every good nurse-midwife–obstetrician relationship is a good supportive backup.

Although I am a great advocate for midwifery, I really think that there are periods in a woman's life where it is probably not the right profession full-time. I still feel very strongly that the mother belongs home with the baby, and that when you have small children, being on call on a full-time basis is not really manageable. As I've said to my daughters, you don't have to accomplish everything in the first decade of work in your profession. Women today are going to live sixty to seventy years, and there are appropriate times for this kind of full-time commitment, and a lot of women go into midwifery after they've had their children.

I wonder sometimes if we as professional women and mothers haven't put a burden on our girls that they must be both, and that it's not just okay to be a mom. I don't know. I'm sitting here with three daughters who are determined to be professional women, and at some point in their lives they will probably sit back and be mothers. I hope I am offering them choices and not handing them a burden.

My oldest daughter is a physician in Boston, and the next one is getting her Ph.D. in clinical psychology, and the next one I hope is going to be a nurse-midwife. She's been in and out of the birth center for years, helping with secretarial stuff and collating materials for the handbook, doing the kinds of things a teenager can do. When I ran into a bout of phlebitis and really had to be off my feet at a time when we only had two nurse-midwives, I had to say to her, "You've got to be my feet." There was no way I could run up and down the stairs of the birth center, and so I brought her along to births with me. She followed me and gave support to women in labor like she'd been doing it for years; I couldn't believe it! Of course, many of the women were her age, and so she really got turned on to it.

I have a very dear friend who is a minister, and we often sit and compare, because, really, our lives are very similar: I'm supporting women in birth, and she's supporting people in death. In both passages, we help people develop the ability to make decisions for themselves around these issues, and this is a new process, and an important one.

With birthing, no matter where it happens, I want women to come through feeling good about themselves and about their new role as a mother so that they can go on to tackle the next aspect, which is rearing the child. And I do believe that most women have this ability. Some women are more comfortable in hospitals and with that image of the health care system as a Big Daddy who is going to take care of it all. They want to be taken care of as opposed to wanting to take charge because so many of them have lost confi-

dence in the ability of their bodies to do this most natural process; this says a lot about our society. We've been through an era in which there was a lot of interest in natural childbirth, and then this epidural [regional anesthesia used to deaden the sensation of contractions during labor or for surgery] epidemic kind of thing starts to take over. The health care system is responsible for much of this. For example, having anesthesia departments solely for OB units often results in having anesthesia pushed on women—they are sold a bill of goods; they are told that this procedure will be a magical cure. They aren't told that epidurals can produce problems which may result in cesarean sections which often would not have been necessary had the drugs not been given.

When a woman does choose to work with a midwife, it's terribly important for her, especially when in labor, to feel the freedom of acceptance from her midwife, to feel that she can say anything she likes. I always tell patients in labor: "Look, when you want me there constantly, you say so. When you don't want me, tell me, you know, feel free. Tell me about all the physical and emotional things you're feeling so I can help you in labor and give you the best deal." It's terribly important for people to know that however they act, however they look, whatever they say to you, they are not going to be judged, that you will accept them. And I don't think that this kind of relationship can be there if you've only seen them once for prenatal care, but it can be established very quickly if you are open with them from the start.

We've had a number of grandmothers attending births, and now that I'm of their age, I'm able to see it through their eyes. And you know most of that generation had the old "knock 'em out, drag 'em out" obstetrics and have not really experienced birth themselves, and so it's wonderful that daughters are willing to share birth experiences with mothers who were denied those experiences.

I've been around a long time, and I've seen nurse-midwives struggle to get where we are today. And I think it's our backgrounds in nursing and our reputation of working within the system that has helped us get this far. I would hate to see anything backtrack because of denial regarding the importance of nursing. Right now there is an acute shortage of nurse-midwives, and it's very dramatic throughout the country. What we need are community-based midwifery programs where women can stay in their own areas to study and be trained.

Common Threads

Each midwife has her own story, her own voice, constituting a strand in a tapestry woven of shared experience. As I gaze at this collective portrait, patterns emerge, common threads that run through the interviews. Some I had sought in my questions; others I could discern only afterward. I see some of these common threads in the midwives' musings on the value of their education, as well as the threads that cross and tangle when midwives disagree about what midwifery education should be. The pattern of their reliance on intuition at birth is beautifully clear, as is the importance of faith and spirituality in the practice of midwifery. A number of midwives drew a parallel between how our culture views women and birth and how it treats the earth. I see the turbulent design made by the midwives' reflections on how their work with birth affects their personal lives: the physical challenges, the dangers of burnout, the stress they feel from the pressures of having to struggle politically for the simple right to practice. But the rewards of being with women at birth are strong, and throughout their stories these women exuded a passion for midwifery and a deep caring for women and birth that give coherence and great beauty to this midwifery tapestry.

Becoming a Midwife:
Educational Paths and Styles

Despite the differing routes through which these midwives entered the field, they all stress the importance of experience, maintaining that the true art of midwifery is learned primarily from birthing women. Even midwives who went through highly academic programs, as did Jo-Anna Rorie, believe their most important lessons came from women themselves:

> I was trained at a high-risk center, and I learned first-rate technology at Yale and at Georgetown. But I learned to be a midwife on my own. And that part of my learning is inside me and connects me to other women, and that's what I draw on to know what is happening with my patients in labor even though I've had no children of my own. That is what lets me know when she's ready to push, or when she's too tired and needs a break, or I need to touch her or I need to walk with her or I need to talk with her—that piece I didn't learn at Yale. That is what I learned year after year after year sitting with and working with women in labor. . . . Now I don't know that you can get that in any educational program.

The components that make up midwifery have been described as a "triangle of skills" and include intellectual skills (theory, critical thinking, and decision making), clinical or manual skills, and personal skills (Page 1993). Where and how these skills are best acquired can vary: intellectual skills can be taught in a classroom setting, but the other two parts of the triangle are best learned through experience. Interpersonal communication, the subtlety of both diagnostic and reassuring touch, helping to ease a baby out, performing medical interventions—all these are complex, interactive skills that don't fit well into classroom learning.

A holistic educational framework integrates these various skills. An important angle to explore is whether or not the way a student is exposed to birth will affect the way she goes on to interpret birth and then to practice midwifery. In the institutional approach to education, the primary emphasis is on biomedical theory; the basic sciences lay the foundation for further theory and practical understanding of birth. During integration, the final phase of nurse-midwifery education, students apply theories and intellectual knowledge to the experience of practice at birth. Edie Wonnell expresses in her interview that the skills and theories acquired during nursing training build a strong foundation for what midwives subsequently learn. But others propose that learning biomedical theories first, before real-life exposure to the com-

plex interactions that occur in the gestalt of birth, gives more validity to theories than to the true experience of birth, which often defies the theories. They argue that communication and intricate hands-on skills are of more value and should be learned first, with theoretical and critical-thinking skills learned later. All three aspects of learning are important; creating a hierarchy of which are most important seems unnecessary, as all three are essential and interlinked.

The midwives interviewed for this book learned their craft either through formal, institutionally based education or through apprenticeship. The difference between these two routes to the practice of midwifery is presently a source of heated debate among midwives. A study of midwives trained through apprenticeship but who then became nurse-midwives revealed an almost universal appreciation of the value of apprenticeship (Bowland, Spindel, and Ventre 1995). Rondi Anderson compared her midwifery apprenticeship to her subsequent academic training and concluded that the mentor relationship that characterizes apprenticeship was invaluable for learning the subtleties of the techniques and art of midwifery. Many times when student nurse-midwives have their first chance at hands-on experience, they are being observed and critiqued by an instructor with whom they may have only a supervisory and evaluative relationship. Confidence is better built from having a trusted relationship with someone; Rondi expressed "the need to have confidence in the birth process in order to really be perceptive."

And yet some nurse-midwifery educators feel that midwifery skills are too complex to be passed on through apprenticeship and that nurse-midwifery needs to be affiliated with universities to maintain its professional status (Roberts 1993). Apprenticeship is often not respected or understood by health care professionals or government authorities. Those who support this model of education have met the challenge of scrutiny with contemporary innovation. The North American Registry of Midwives (NARM) national certification program described in the Introduction has analyzed the components of the core competencies that must be provided by midwifery education and has made a detailed breakdown of the physical and theoretical skills needed to safely practice midwifery. This process is similar to what educational programs within accredited institutions define and evaluate as "learning objectives." It has been tailored for the individual's use in her apprenticeship setting. This is in essence what underlies the theory of mastery learning, the cornerstone of nurse-midwifery education:

> Mastery learning differs from traditional learning classroom practices
> in calling for special attention to the individual student's progress and
> careful matching of teacher activities to the student's learning needs.
> Research and anecdotal reports of the use of mastery learning at all
> educational levels overwhelmingly support the value of mastery learn-
> ing for increasing individual student learning. (Decker 1990)

Examining the attitudes of lay midwives who went through a CNM
program, Linda Walsh questions what makes education different from educational credentials. Lay midwives often entered their CNM programs with
significant life experience and then had to interact with educators who had
worked only within academic and hospital settings. Only one in five nurse-
midwifery educators had ever worked outside of a hospital setting. These
students also entered with a firm idea of what midwifery should be, an idea
that was often in conflict with the medical paradigm that influences nurse-
midwifery instructors' definition of normal. (For example, a CNM considers
the routine use of technologies like ultrasound and electronic fetal monitoring, and surgical interventions like episiotomy to be normal). One of the
nurse-midwifery educators' complaints was that lay midwives were difficult to
"socialize into the hierarchy of hospital practices" (Walsh and Jaspar 1990).
Rondi Anderson's story provides another example of this struggle.

This concern over how midwives learn midwifery was expressed throughout the interviews. Many felt that the process of education is as important as
(and indeed affects) what is learned, just as the process of birth is important
and affects both mother and baby. Connie Breece condemns the demeaning
treatment she felt she received as a nursing student. The midwifery model of
education is based on belief rather than doubt, on creating a nurturing environment for the student who is unfolding into a midwife:

> Education conducted on the connected model would help women
> toward community, power, and integrity. Such an education could
> facilitate the development of women's minds and spirits . . . rather
> than retarding, arresting, or even reversing their growth. (Belenky et
> al. 1986:228)

The research on women's ways of knowing shows that the use of conflict as
an impetus to growth is also inherent in the learning process, but women do
not usually see situations where they were aggressively challenged in their
thinking as positive learning experiences (Belenky et al. 1986).

Independent midwifery educator Elizabeth Davis was surprised by the
insecurity of new nurse-midwifery graduates from her area who called her for

advice regarding starting a practice. She expected them to be asking her for some of the nitty-gritty organizational details of getting a midwifery practice going, yet they were most interested in how she found the confidence to attend homebirths and even to practice midwifery. Davis expressed a concern for students who emerge from programs with little faith in the normalcy of birth and without the self-confidence needed to react quickly in emergencies (Davis 1992).

Many nurse-midwives are now trained in tertiary-care centers that are organized around handling high-risk and complicated situations, and they, like medical residents, see a disproportionate number of abnormal births. Connie Breece felt that her work at a large inner-city hospital exposed her to such a broad spectrum of complications and outcomes that it gave her confidence to deal with problems that she would face in the future. Many nurse-midwives insist that midwives trained by apprenticeship lack skills essential for dealing with complications they may face. Candace Whitridge looks at the opposite side of that coin:

> I think that many of these midwives are going to births carrying a great deal of fear with them. I don't think fear should be a part of midwifery care—certainly vigilance and respect for something big and knowing that nature's not perfect, but that's not fear. That's a respect that you bring with you so that you are really watchful. I'm not sure that this is happening in most educational programs since they are based at tertiary-care centers. How can you not become afraid of birth when all you are seeing are women with premature births and hemorrhages and multiple problems based on clientele who have social and medical factors that make birth difficult for them? I think that your grounding should be in normal births first, and from there bring your understanding of that to skillful care for women with special needs. (Interview with Whitridge, 1992)

Penny Armstrong tries to teach midwifery preceptors how to "demystify and put words to the art of midwifery." Attention to adult learning processes and styles has been brought to many midwifery educational programs, especially those that are community-based. These programs (both nurse and direct entry) acknowledge the importance of life-learning to the practice of midwifery, experience that younger students can gain only as they mature. These programs rely on the student to take responsibility for her own learning with the support and guidance of a teacher (Silverton 1996). Edie Wonnell pointed out that it is important to make community-based programs available because many women enter the field of midwifery after having

children themselves. While most midwives agree that it is important to make midwifery education more readily available, the move within nurse-midwifery has been toward masters' level education, not so much to increase midwives' skills but "as a way of increasing the elitism of the profession and, consequently, its political power." One nurse-midwifery educator bemoans this trend:

> Where is the wisdom, then, in adopting a requirement that may deter access to the profession, particularly if the women who are deterred are similar to the ones we serve—women with families, women of color, women of vulnerable populations? To better serve these women, we need to recruit, not restrict, women from these backgrounds. (Lichtman 1996)

Others who support the notion of keeping midwifery education as close as possible to the community do so because it helps to foster "less hierarchical division between the professional and the lay person so that the community also takes more responsibility for its own health. As well, the midwives are constantly reminded that they are there to serve the community which provides the school to them in the first place" (COMBS 1992).

An essential question remains: How can midwives teach and pass on to others a midwifery philosophy of birth through educational programs within a culture that depends on a medical model of birth? In her survey of educators, Linda Walsh sees a trend toward teaching obstetrics rather than midwifery. She notes the danger in this approach:

> To define a student's ability to move into the role of the nurse-midwife by placing emphasis on the ability to practice using medically based indicators serves only to place midwifery increasingly under the domain of medicine. The almost total reliance on research as defined by a scientific model that is masculine and mechanistic in nature limits development and application of knowledge in our field. (Walsh and Jaspar 1990:212)

I think that only through conscious awareness of and resistance to the medical paradigm can midwifery survive and flourish. In holistic midwifery, information and treatment are drawn from numerous disciplines and approaches to health, including herbalism, homeopathy, massage, and acupuncture. Learning how these systems of knowledge can intersect or be used sequentially can support a broad base of knowledge that does not totally rely on biomedical theories as "authoritative knowledge" (Jordan 1993). When midwifery education is based on the medical model of education, then teach-

ing makes exclusive use of objective language (with linear logic), which reifies the authority of science (Hubbard 1992). Barbara Duden (1993) describes what she sees as a destructive alienation and depersonalization of women in the scientific drive to delve deeper and deeper into the woman's body for knowledge. This could be countered by incorporating Eastern modes of educational inquiry into education: models such as Tibetan medicine, which is based on a more integrated holistic model of the body, one in which any part of the body is treated in a way that recognizes that every other part will also be affected. The importance of connection would then be highlighted, instead of the medical model's separation of the body into parts—a separation that is supported by logical, sequential language and that dictates subsequent diagnoses and treatment.

In contrast to medical education, which fosters in students the idea that they "master" a body of knowledge, I would hope that we could invite midwifery students into the never-ending mysteries of the process of birth. Just as true scientists are invited to question preconceived assumptions and look for undiscovered truth, we could encourage students to question accepted institutional or medical authority, developing their own internal authority instead.

With the recent development of national certification of direct-entry, or independent, midwives, it has been vital to define what constitutes a midwifery knowledge base as distinct from a medical model of obstetrical knowledge. It is important that midwives be aware that theirs is a unique profession based on a different philosophy of birth than that of the dominant medical model. In medicine, the most trusted information is that obtained from external diagnostic technologies. In contrast, a deep trust in the value of intuition—the knowing that arises from deep inside one's being—is integral to midwifery practice and philosophy.

Intuition in Midwifery

Intuition underlies the art of midwifery and yet is not highly valued in our culture, so it was interesting to me how often this common thread came up in midwives' stories. I posed no questions regarding intuition in my interviews; yet it was named by many midwives as a skill they use at difficult births. Jill Breen put it this way:

> Our standards have to be accountable to our values, not to the values of traditional medical practice in this country. For example, with the training of midwives . . . let's decide how a midwife should be tested,

and let's test her that way. Let's not kiss up to the standards of the medical profession in order to satisfy them that we are competent. Let's satisfy *ourselves* that we are competent. Intuition is often what makes us smart, what makes us do the work best, what makes us able to pick up problems earlier than anyone else and therefore deal with them more effectively.

In a recent study, midwife Elizabeth Davis and anthropologist Robbie Davis-Floyd (1996) note that for homebirth midwives, intuition often constitutes "authoritative knowledge"—knowledge on the basis of which decisions are made and actions taken (Jordan 1993)—as midwives often give higher priority to intuition than to rational, linear thinking when making decisions at births. "The deep value that they place on connection, in the context of their holistic model of birth and health care, leads them to listen and follow their inner voice during birth, rather than operating only according to protocols and standard parameters for 'normal birth'" (Davis and Davis-Floyd 1996). Jeannine Parvati Baker speaks of learning to trust her intuition from her own birth experiences. Anne Frye says: "My intuition at birth has more to do with tuning in to birthing energy on some subtle level, just allowing myself to be, and paying attention to how I'm feeling as I listen to the heart tones or how I'm feeling when I'm palpating a baby."

To demonstrate how intuition can help with decision making, nurse-midwife Tina Guy tells a story about bringing a homebirth woman into the hospital during labor even though everything measurable had checked out at home; after arriving at the hospital, the laboring woman developed a problem, confirming Tina's underlying sense of the situation. Midwives often refer to this as "listening to their gut"—intuition as a felt sensation. Jeannine Parvati Baker and Toni House both commented that we can learn more about how to use our intuition by paying attention to nature, and our "animal selves." Elizabeth Davis also encourages the development of intuition in decision making. She feels that she uses intuition to show her how to act, based on the pieces of information she gathers using her rational abilities.

Ina May Gaskin learned from her physician mentor to trust a mother's sense about her child even if nothing is immediately discernible. Through "intuitive flashes," midwives can develop "tricks" for helping women in labor. She feels that

> the subconscious mind is able to pick up signals too subtle to be perceived by the conscious mind, and the mind can apprehend the gestalt, which may surface in the form of intuition, a hunch, or a

dream. It should not be surprising that a deep level of insight about the subtleties of the labor process can come to the practitioner whose presence during labor is uninterrupted. (Gaskin 1996:296)

Intuition may be too slippery to be pinned down, quantified, and tested, yet its importance is acknowledged within the national midwifery certification process: "We recognize that midwifery requires attributes and skills which defy measurement" (North American Registry of Midwives 1996). MANA includes intuition within the essential core competencies for midwifery practice: "Midwives synthesize clinical observations, theoretical knowledge, intuitive assessment and spiritual awareness as components of a competent decision-making process" (Midwives' Alliance of North America 1994). And yet, if intuition cannot be measured, can it be taught? The struggle to have intuitive authority valued will inevitably be ongoing in a culture that values the authority of institutions, men, and linear, rational knowledge over the authoritative knowledge of women, birth, the body, and the individual (Davis-Floyd 1992; Jordan 1993).

Faith and Spirituality in Midwifery

Spiritual awareness was another recurring theme, a central feature of midwives' lives and practice. Some midwives are devoutly religious in a conventional sense. Sister Angela Murdaugh is one obvious example, as she is a member of a religious order that is called upon to give health care service. She is a witness to God working through her at births:

> You see miracles happen in your hands and you become faith-filled. You know *you* didn't do it. Your hands moved, but something else did that. . . . I call the difficult births "three Hail Mary deliveries"— yes, definitely you have faith to fall back on.

Shafia Munroe, a Muslim, recounts learning a special prayer from the Koran for difficult births and attests to the importance of praying at normal births too. She warns her clients that she may pray out loud at births in Arabic and remembers how midwives in the South got down on their knees and prayed when they arrived at a woman's house.

Faith Gibson talks about how nursing used to be considered a religious vocation and how her work has always been a part of her spiritual life. Faith practices legally now in California under the religious exemptions clause. She will attend the homebirths of any couple who will sign papers attesting to

their belief that birth is a spiritual act. She sees her midwifery as a three-way partnership with the couple and God. She describes herself as being co-creative with God and relies on prayer to give her the inner strength to handle the difficult situations and decisions she has to make at births.

Gladys Milton consults with God when confronted with situations where she is concerned about the progress of a laboring mother. Gladys also prays before each birth and has seen the miracle of prayer serve her in times of crisis.

Other midwives who profess no active involvement with a particular religion also talk of their reliance on spirit or something outside of themselves to guide them in midwifery. Kaye Kanne says:

> I usually think of me as more than one—the guides are there. . . . Sometimes I get a rush of fear, and I have to distinguish where it's coming from. . . . And then I use prayer—I guess you would call it prayer, meditation—just letting go and saying, "Okay, whatever, just let me know what it is I need to do." It works, it works really well. . . . I couldn't do midwifery if I didn't think there was a higher purpose to what I am doing.

Connie Breece feels the need to protect the sacred space of birth, which is also how Mary Cooper sees her role. Reinterpreting childbirth as a sacred event highlights the spiritual nature of midwifery. Analyzing the practices and writings of three independent midwives and authors (Rahima Baldwin, Ina May Gaskin, and Elizabeth Davis), Kathryn Rabuzzi frames much of their work in terms of spirituality and describes the importance and intensity of community shared during birth: "Communion at its holiest, this sharing of the creation of new life clearly manifests the sacred dimension of childbearing. It is a very important gynocentric vision of childbirth" (Rabuzzi 1994:86).

Jeannine Parvati Baker's spiritual practice of yoga is integral to her practice of midwifery; she interprets the birth experience as primarily a spiritual event:

> You recognize that this baby is participating in the birth, and in my language I say that the Goddess is coming through me in birth, in this transpersonal experience. That is why ecstasy flows through me and during birth I connect with every woman who has ever given birth and ever will. At that moment when I have a baby emerging through me—I know we're two beings, but we look like we're one. It's a profound spiritual experience.

Jeannine describes her midwifery as a type of shamanism that involves the transformation of the psychological and spiritual nature of the woman and

her family. She blends the wisdom and tradition of psychology and spirituality in her approach, considering birth an archetypal event, the birth being the death of the maiden as the mother is born.

This spiritual dimension of birth is strikingly different from what is found in the predominant mechanistic model of birth in hospitals. Looking for a language of birth in our society, sociologist Robbie Pfeufer Kahn (1995) comments: "The social context created by obstetrics denudes childbirth of the sacred. Major Western religious systems that contribute to the cultural context of birth (which could give women access to the spiritual) are male constructs." Not surprisingly, Kahn continues, where culture and society offer such inhospitable environments, women "lack a language" for spiritual experience in childbirth. In contrast, the midwives in these narratives invite an exploration into the spiritual nature of birth.

Ecofeminism in Midwifery: *"Women of Earth, Take Back Your Birth"*

This slogan found on a bumper sticker popular with midwives expresses the connection between how we attend to women at birth and how we attend to the earth. A number of the midwives I interviewed spoke of this awareness in their work—an awareness not shared by all members of the larger feminist community. There has been a split within feminist thought concerning childbirth and the female body:

> For some, feminism has meant a rejection of traditional female roles, so tied to birth and breastfeeding—a rejection that has often led them to free themselves from the entrapment of those biological processes. For others, feminism means a celebration, a "re-membering," of the female body and its organicity, and a re-claiming of the value and importance of birthgiving, breastfeeding, and childcare. (Davis-Floyd 1994)

The social movement of ecofeminism recognizes the potential that women have through childbearing (including breastfeeding and menstruation) to acknowledge and celebrate that we are *of nature*. As childbearers, women are the ones closest to being instructed by newborns about the necessity of nurturing, but these embodied lessons can extend to anyone exposed to infants. "The culture of the just-born influences adults and older children of both genders and can prompt grown-ups to enact social change" (Kahn 1995:138).

Candace Whitridge's analogy between her work as an organic farmer

and her work as a midwife is one of the most obvious and extensive references to ecofeminism in this collection of narratives. Jeannine Parvati Baker sees her work as an effort to heal the earth, "because unless we bring in more babies that are able to be in resonance with the earth and feel connected to life, our planet is not long going to allow two-leggeds to continue our existence here."

Sister Angela Murdaugh observes that the Mexican women whose births she attends still have a close relationship to the earth through their agricultural work, and that they have a parallel respect for birth. In contrast, Therese Stallings laments that most American women are disconnected from and distrustful of their bodies, making it hard for them to trust the birth process and thereby trust midwives. By working with women in dance and drumming, she hopes that she can help women to discover fuller awareness and respect for their bodies, in turn allowing them to find power and satisfaction in their birthing experience.

Connie Breece describes herself as a planetarian:

> I don't think of myself as being from a particular country. I think of myself as someone who's living on the earth, and that there are universal forces that guide us all along, and we're in a place in the universe that's gotten pretty out of touch with that. I think part of the work is to move people back toward what those forces are. And there are few places in daily life where you get to watch them at work as much as you do at a birth.

Penny Armstrong thinks that the disintegration of women's birthing culture is akin to our disregard for the natural patterns of the world:

> The experience that I had from working with the Amish showed me that the farther you get away from the earth, the farther you take birth away. I think that each layer, each hospital floor takes you farther away from the earth, then you lose the connections to the rhythms and the cycles. You can't reproduce that in a plastic environment. . . .
>
> I don't know what is holding women back from using midwives except that I think there is a cultural imperative to separate women from birthing, to separate families. I think there is a cultural imperative to separate us from the earth from which we get all of our powers and from our animal instincts. And I think that that movement is much more potentially dangerous for us as practicing midwives than all the laws of any state or country.

Ina May Gaskin sees the inherent role of midwives as peacekeepers and community workers, making them both political and spiritual activists in a very

practical way. Her efforts to create a community supportive of both birthing and dying express her hope that as a people we can become more compassionate, designing health care that responds to the needs of people and not just profits: "I'm convinced that if we make a nice place for babies to land, it will be a nice place for the rest of us."

Burnout

Midwives share with other caregivers the tendency to experience emotional burnout. In choosing midwives to interview, I tried to pick those who are still actively attending births, but I included some who are not so that this book would also represent the many midwives who continue to serve women in other ways. The lifestyle of a midwife is full of physical challenges, including lack of sleep, unpredictable hours, and accommodating the various awkward positions that a woman can take during childbirth. But it is the emotional demands that create the greatest amount of stress for midwives. Kaye Kanne articulates the need for a strong support system. Having time to be with her family and setting limits regarding when she is available to talk with her clients in nonemergencies has helped her keep her practice from taking over her life. Needs for support and for time away from the intensity of midwifery practice were voiced a number of times. Many nurse-midwives have found that sharing with midwifery partners the burden of being on call has helped them keep a balance in their lives, to relieve some of the stress of always being available.

Sister Angela Murdaugh talked about how people have different psychological strengths:

> I've had partners fizzle or go on to do even bigger things. Extraneous things can cause burnout. Sacrifices are necessary. Being a midwife is stressful. Every day you're at work, making decisions. It's not rote. At some point, you need a break. Midwives get into foolish situations occasionally, like getting into practice by themselves.

Edie Wonnell comments that there are times in a woman's life when it may not be right for her to practice as a midwife, particularly if she has young children. Wonnell is concerned that the pressure for young women to be professional and have families at the same time can be terribly stressful. She feels that there should be time at different points of our lives to do both. Candace Whitridge felt strongly that

there are midwives out there whose lives are screaming at them to stop practicing right now. They need to put things on hold for a while, especially when it is so discordant in their families. We hold in our midwifery practice this ideal of integration of family and love and birth, and yet it's a paradox when our lives are in shambles around us. I have met some midwives who I know are clinging to their midwifery because they think it is feeding them in some way that sustains them. And I think to myself, "You need to let go of this right now." Sometimes what happens is that they're becoming the indispensable midwife. Which we have to be very careful that we don't do. As midwives, we're notorious for substituting as the external factor that women are dependent on. If you in fact have got people so strongly doing birth themselves, and you have truly become this little assistant for them, if people can't even remember who was there at their birth, then I think you have done a pretty good job.

The challenge of maintaining a solo midwifery practice is one that wears out many midwives. While defending the importance of having this solo type of practice, Penny Armstrong also shares her story of burnout, comparing it with the grief process:

> I remember thinking that I was dead, spiritually, that the part of me that just rebounds—which is an important part of my being—was gone. Not to overemphasize the negative part of it, but very few people are honest about the cost of this kind of work. No one wants to hear about it either. Everybody wants you to be a hero. They want you to be what they need you to be. . . . People have taken it really personally that I am tired.

Penny did return to midwifery, first into a group practice, where she worked one weekend out of a month and then as a midwifery educator. This is the path many midwives eventually take—becoming educators, lecturers, or administrators. The definition of midwife then expands to include those who contribute to midwifery in ways other than attending births, a notion that contradicts currently held views:

> The underlying assumption . . . is that nurse-midwifery is no more than its practice. If you don't practice, you are not counted among the ranks of "active" midwives. Thus, you lose your identity and acceptance as a midwife. This may serve as a means of clarifying midwives' identity to outsiders, but it negates the belief that midwifery is a philosophy as well as a professional practice: a belief in women and their families, a respect for their being and their potential, and a

commitment to their health care that stresses the support of health, normalcy, and family bonds in a holistic way. (Murphy 1987:121)

Legal threat and harassment have also pushed many midwives to burnout and to leaving midwifery entirely. One example of this is the choice that the midwife who wished to remain anonymous made after our interview. After a number of years of practicing illegally, she finally succumbed to the pressure and retired. Many other midwives move into nurse-midwifery to have protection from harassment even if it means being unable to practice in their preferred setting or style.

Raven Lang speaks of midwives losing "chi," a vital energy force recognized in Chinese medicine, at each birth. "The work of midwifery is so elemental, so taking of the essence of who you are" (Reichman 1988:15). However, Raven was a single parent struggling to make her way through acupuncture school when she came to that conclusion, and she had few personal resources to fill up her own well of energy and well-being. The rewards for the demanding work of midwifery must be available and truly taken in by the midwife to balance the constant stress of being available to women during the psychically, physically, and emotionally demanding time of childbirth.

Political Struggles

The political struggles that midwives face both inside and outside of the system emerge from their personal narratives as being the most stressful part of their work, countering the rewarding, satisfying part of the profession. Trudy Cox told of how these unrelenting pressures pushed her to the edge:

> It wasn't the births. It was the schizophrenic life of what I did inside that birthing room, under tremendous pressure, and what I had to do on the outside of that door to fend off the [medical] community and the nurses. . . . That door was like a lid on a pressure cooker. I couldn't function with the staff at the hospital. There was an unbelievable amount of conflict and pressure, and with the lack of support it was very destructive to me. You know the average working life of a certified nurse-midwife is only ten years. And it's not the patients, it's the system.

Although midwives agree that midwifery should be available to all women, there is much disagreement on how this should be done. Some feel it is essential that midwifery be integrated into the health care system, whereas others feel it is imperative for some form of midwifery to stay outside the

system or on its fringes. Because of increased visibility, financial reimbursement, and dependable backup relationships for collaboration or transfer of care, it is easier for women to have access to midwives when the midwives work within the system. Yet in an institution constructed along the medical model, the problem of primary accountability surfaces—should the midwife be accountable to women or to the powers that be (Kirkham 1996)?

In an ideal world, professional practice and accountability would be based on experiential wisdom (personal and collective) used in respectful service to the individual. Given the current reality of the inequality of power and privilege in our society, as defined by economic class, gender, and race, however, financial and resource allocations (as well as psychological privileges) are distributed unevenly. With the shift to managed care, changes in access to and reimbursement of health services put midwifery in a precarious position. Perseverance and creativity are needed to ensure that midwives will remain accessible to women who want their care.

The difficulty of midwifery's surviving and flourishing results not only from political and financial forces outside of the profession but also from dissension within the profession. Different sectors of midwives have conflicting views regarding the parameters of midwifery and even regarding who should be called a midwife and what her education should be. The argument over who is the real midwife is pointless, as midwives from the three historically separate and unique branches all successfully attend women at birth, even though they may differ greatly in education, skills, and the settings in which they practice. (See Rooks 1997 for a comprehensive review of outcomes of midwife-attended births in diverse settings.)

When a fledgling midwife looks at the midwifery news list on the Internet for help in deciding which path to take to become a "real midwife," she might also ask herself what kinds of women, with what kinds of values, she ultimately wants to serve. The midwives in this collection express such different attitudes and experiences of being with women at birth that the reader can quickly come to understand why midwives who practice at one end of the spectrum are sometimes unable to recognize as colleagues and sisters those at the other end (DeVries 1992).

The American College of Nurse-Midwives (ACNM) wants to limit the use of the term *midwife* in the following way: "The ACNM believes that any individual who uses the title 'midwife' should be registered or licensed at the state or jurisdictional level, should be held to a defined and verifiable level of education and competence, and should participate in professional activities

designed to assure current knowledge and expertise" (American College of Nurse-Midwives 1996). So in their eyes, all those midwives who practice outside of the system's regulation would not be considered midwives but "birth attendants."

Helen Varney Burst more specifically explores the conflict within the profession of nurse-midwifery regarding who practices "real midwifery." Burst encourages CNMs to consider that in all the various settings, they are practicing midwifery:

> "Real" midwifery is not determined by the locale or by medical and obstetrical normalcy. "Real" midwifery is not determined by whether the woman is not in stirrups, has no limit on her visitors, does not get moved to a delivery room, or can eat and drink during labor.
>
> "Real" midwifery is what we do wherever the woman is. It is how we approach the woman and include her and her family in the process. It is the application of all our knowledge, skills, and beliefs within a situation. It is how we facilitate normal, natural processes and foster participatory decision making. It is how we can be creative when there are restrictions placed upon us.
>
> *Real* midwifery is "with woman" wherever she may be, in whatever circumstances she may be in, in whatever condition her pregnancy, in whatever health care system. (Burst 1990:191)

It is this definition of midwifery that includes the various women I interviewed; however, this inclusive definition of *midwife* does not extend to how midwifery as a profession is viewed. The concept of "professional" continues to be debated, defined, and described in various ways within midwifery. Do the members of a profession openly share their specialized knowledge with those who receive their care, thereby empowering them, or are they elitist, withholding and protecting their knowledge from others? As Jill Breen puts it: "I don't want to be a professional who's up above them, that's why I call myself a 'community midwife.' I want to be on an equal footing with my clients."

Two aspects of these conflicting views are often debated by midwives: simple mastery of skills versus using those skills to become part of an institution that holds power within a society. Midwives are particularly sensitive to this issue because when they practice within the health care system, they are accountable to a group that holds some of the highest economic and political power in this country—the medical profession—yet midwives' service and original allegiance is to a group that traditionally has the least amount of financial and political power in this country, namely, women and children,

and especially women of color. New Zealand midwives have articulated a vision of working in partnership with women: "Partnership does not restrict a profession but enhances and empowers all women's status including midwives. Partnership includes professionalism but tempers elitism. Partnership ensures that a profession looks outward at the reasons why it exists rather than turning inward and becoming self-serving" (Guilliland 1993:785). The anonymous midwife echoes this when she says: "I've always felt that they [midwives] should be handmaidens to women and not to the system, and not to the establishment and not to doctors and medical schools, but their service should be to women."

Nurse-midwifery faces its own struggles with defining and maintaining its identity. Some CNMs believe they are able to exist only with the support of obstetricians who are responding to consumer pressure (Lichtman 1988). They feel that the care they give is only as good as their backup. CNMs are sometimes seen by clients as part of the medical staff. As one midwife pointed out, she has been called "Dr. Ronnie" (Lichtman 1988). Lewis Mehl warns that midwifery is in a problematic place when the medical residents he works with ask why the hospital bothers to have midwives when they do nothing differently from the residents (Mehl and Madronna 1993/1994).

Henci Goer points out the danger of midwifery becoming indistinguishable from the medical system: "Because the obstetric model holds sway, the acceptance of midwifery into the mainstream has a price: co-optation. Enormous social, political, and economic pressures constrain midwives from practicing midwifery (as opposed to obstetrics)" (Goer 1995:300).

Most of the time midwives still lose in the conflict with doctors, as doctors hold places of power and authority in our institutional structures— insurance companies, legislatures, hospital boards. Midwives who work in hospital-based services struggle to give the care that the philosophy of midwifery is based on: personal attention, educating the pregnant woman, honoring her individuality, and developing a trusting relationship through continuity of care (Goer 1995). When forced to practice in ways that disregard the woman's individual needs and encourage an indiscriminate use of technology, midwives are reinforcing the society's dictates of appropriate gender roles—ones that devalue the woman (Burst and Vosler 1993):

> The relationship of nurse-midwifery to the establishment is fraught
> with contradictions and tensions. The insistence of nurse-midwifery
> throughout its history to be in a relationship with medicine by func
> tioning in a health care system that provides for physician consulta-

tion, collaboration, and referral has had two effects. One effect has been the intended one of assuring physician involvement when needed for the benefit of the patient. Another effect, however, has been the negative one of placing nurse-midwives in a position of dependency upon the physician. This dependency gives the physician ultimate power and control both over whether a nurse-midwife can practice in a given community and over the practice itself. (Burst and Vosler 1993)

This power is wielded through denial of hospital privileges, insurance reimbursement, and prescriptive authority. Raymond DeVries (1992) proposes that the way an occupational group gains power, or acceptance, in American society is to emphasize the risk involved in life events: the greater the risk and uncertainty, the more value and power the profession has. He points out that we have shifted ultimate power from our spiritual leaders to the legal and medical professions because we consider our material possessions and bodies more important than our souls. He feels that midwives have less of a chance to acquire a respected place within modern medical systems because of their emphasis on being the experts in the normal and the low risk. Because midwives try to reduce the emphasis on risk and fear in birth and instead to value the inherent normalcy of birth and the power of the birthing woman (neither of which is valued by the wider society), DeVries suspects that they may be unable to gain credibility as professionals in our society.

While many nurse-midwives are working inside of hospitals to set a high standard of nurturant care for indigent women, the predominant way that homebirth midwifery affects the society at large is not so much through those few who experience homebirth care by independent midwives but through how those few affect mainstream obstetrics. Therese Stallings talks about keeping the tiny flame of direct-entry midwifery and homebirth alive to preserve another possibility for women, even though for most it is just there as a conceptual space. Paradigm shifts are usually generated at the edges of society, not by those who are in the dominant core (Davis-Floyd 1992). This is exemplified in the new wave of birth centers in hospitals that advertise "just like home, only safer." Hospitals concerned with increased competition have recognized the appeal of the joyful, family-centered, and woman-empowering aspects of homebirth and try to incorporate those concepts into an institutional setting that society sees as safe. Because homebirth midwives offer an attractive alternative, the doctors in the mainstream are challenged to make medical, hospitalized birth more humane (Wertz and Wertz 1989; Sakala 1993).

Perhaps midwives will survive to serve only those women and families

who share a different belief and system of values like that articulated by MANA (see Appendix A) rather than those who abide by and try to fit into the dominant system. This may be what Trudy Cox refers to when she says that midwives are revolutionary and that the only way midwifery can really flourish in this country is through basic social change. Therese Stallings, like other midwives, feels that women need to have the confidence in their bodies (or be "re-embodied") to have the faith to give birth with midwives who feel that the natural authority of birth belongs to women. The MANA Statement of Values and Ethics (Appendix A) expresses a type of female reality—one that acknowledges the importance of relationship, the connection of mother and child as an "inseparable and interdependent whole." It supports the notion that the mysterious nature of birth is something that women and midwives strive to understand and work with, but not to control. Death is not the enemy or the end, but an accepted part of life. Taking the view that "birth is as safe as life gets" incorporates the acceptance of death. The process of birth as inherent to the dignity and worth of women is considered as important as the ultimate "product" or outcome of the pregnancy and birth. The inherent value of intuitive thinking and of connection are core to the nature of midwifery (Midwives' Alliance of North America 1992).

In a society that does not currently support these values, midwifery acts as a catalyst for social change, one baby at a time, through the care of one mother, one family at a time. Faith Gibson sees her midwifery as a service that she offers in penance for the hospital maternity care she participated in, which she felt was barbaric and unethical. She encourages midwives to use the skills they learn from being with women at birth to "midwife the system." I have often thought about how the violence that is perpetrated against women in our society is reflected in the way women are treated when they give birth. Arizika Razak describes how the essence of birth is a metaphor upon which our culture could be based:

> The reversal of cultural attitudes of rape and rapaciousness is of fundamental importance to the issue of our societal health. Put quite simply, healthy human beings do not rape each other. But we also need new paradigms that articulate positive human interaction and functioning. We need models that are more inclusive and holistic. We need paradigms that are nurturing. We need models based on human cycles of growth and change, not mechanistic interactions of stasis and motion. I would like to propose that birth is such a universal and central aspect of human existence that it can serve as the nucleus around which to build a paradigm of positive human interaction. . . .

Let the shared experience of birth reclaim the human soul. (Razak 1990)

Midwives who have been engaged in political work see how problems of our society stem from the struggles in our individual family histories. They strive for change by working within the microcosm of pregnancy, birth, and postpartum parenting to help promote health and healing for women, for children, and for families.

Rewards for the Midwife

The counterbalance to burnout as a result of selfless service is found in the rewards of midwifery and childbirth. The midwives I spoke with shared some of the many gifts that they received in their practice. In her book *Sensitive Midwifery* (1987), Caroline Flint takes the whole first chapter to remind midwives of the ways in which to take care of and cherish themselves. She gives little tips about keeping a special "lovely box" to store letters and photos of special times when you have been appreciated. She advises on building and nurturing relationships that are supportive to oneself, and giving oneself nurturing self-care through relaxation and participation in activities that are pleasurable and renewing. She insists that

> for midwives to be able to love, cherish and care for women through-out pregnancy, labour, the puerperium, midwives need to be loved, cherished and cared for themselves. We work in an emotional mine-field. . . . For us to practice as true midwives, for us to learn to be close to women and have empathy with them, we must first get to know and love the woman who is nearest to us—ourselves. (Flint 1987:1)

One of the rewards that a midwife receives is found in her relationship with the birthing woman and her family. Candace Whitridge spoke of the pleasure she got from watching children in her community who recognize her role in their births grow into adulthood. Midwives see the tremendous growth women achieve during pregnancy and birth and their increasing personal empowerment. Midwives who work in situations where they have little continuity of care miss out on this reward more than those who can witness the evolution of the family. It is easier for a midwife to maintain connection and provide support for a laboring woman if she knows her in the context of her life. Candace reflects on the importance of story-telling and getting to know a woman well during the course of her prenatal care to be able to best help her in the demanding time of labor.

Anne Frye feels that midwifery has helped her to grow as a person:

> It is not a superficial kind of job—it offers me the challenge of being
> in new situations all the time because each birth is new. When things
> get too stressful from dealing with on-the-edge situations, I've often
> joked that I should just be a clerk at Woolworth's, but I could never
> do that. I get bored too easily. Midwifery affords me enough intellec-
> tual challenge and other stimulation to keep me interested. Over the
> years I have been drawn to different aspects of what our work as
> midwives entails; it is so multifaceted. Each birth is unique, and it
> requires you to be a detective, a clinician, and a counselor.

Having a viable business is another reward for some midwives and has
been an underlying motivation for some independent midwives to move into
nurse-midwifery. Many lay midwives began more from a spiritual sense of
service, providing care as a sister or friend would, their motivation later shifting to a more financial or career-oriented stance. The demands of an active
midwifery practice preclude the former type of relationship, however, with
the necessary reward being increased financial stability. Kaye Kanne believes
this shift to being compensated adequately for her work helped how her family felt about her work. Raven Lang described her change from just helping at
births without payment to the realization that she needed to be compensated
for her work:

> Somehow we must have something given back to us in return for our
> work for our community. They have got to fix your car, put on the
> roof, or pay you the money for your service. I did it for nothing
> [back] then. I did it for a hug and a kiss. Now I charge one thousand
> dollars. (Reichman 1988:16)

Along with financial rewards goes the value of recognition. Jesusita Aragon made sure that I noticed on the wall the awards she had received from
the community. Jeannine Parvati Baker notes being nominated in the *International Women's Who's Who* for her contributions to medicine. Gladys Milton also shared her pleasure at being given the Sage Femme Award at
MANA. These awards are symbolic of being accepted and recognized for
hard work that so often goes unnoticed or, worse, is derided and devalued by
the society at large.

Another reward that midwives spoke of was being able to share in the
intimacy and miracle of birth. There is a special gift in being one of the first to
receive a newborn into your hands. Elizabeth Gilmore and Jeannine Parvati

Baker, along with others, feel that midwives need to realize that they are going to births for themselves, not just for the mother and family. Baker says:

> It's really important that we know that we are midwives because we are being selfish. I am involved in midwifery for selfish motives. It's because I want more babies born on this planet who are deeply loved and bonded to their source, who are gentle beings, who are healthy, so that my children will be able to find suitable mates and I can have healthy grandchildren and then the earth can sustain itself. . . . It's not altruism that has drawn me to this. . . . I'm involved in midwifery still for soul-making, for my own reclamation of who I am. . . . I'm in the process of being all of who I can be, too, and that is through the relationship that I have with the woman giving birth.

Finally, Therese Stallings articulates the gift of the miracle of babies:

> As a midwife, a feminine part of myself was evoked. A newborn baby hasn't done anything, and yet I love newborn babies. They are probably my favorite part about midwifery—they're just fresh and I would have unconditional love for a newborn baby. . . . The baby just is, and that love *is* because of that essence, not because of what somebody's done to prove that they are lovable. And then I asked myself, Can I treat myself that way?

And I hope that the anonymous midwife, who has since stopped practicing, still treasures the rewards of midwifery as she saw them:

> You see a birth, and as most births unfold, you've watched magic, you've watched God, you've watched miracles, you've watched nature—you've seen it all! Right there before your eyes—and have been able to participate in it in a very special way. It comes with a price, but it's a pretty wonderful thing to walk around with.

Afterword

Visions for the Future of Midwifery

Again and again I have been asked during this project: What about the future of midwifery? The dynamic changes in health care had not really begun in earnest at the beginning of my interviewing process, so I didn't ask this question specifically, although considering the interest in it today I now wish I had. After listening to the varied voices of these midwives, however, I feel that the ability to hold paradox and complexity lightly and with grace is essential to envisioning a future for midwifery in which its essence remains uncompromised while access to it is increased.

On the subject of creating a sustainable future for midwifery, the midwives I interviewed voiced the following views: (1) all women need access to midwives throughout their life cycles, as midwives offer not only perinatal care, but also care during puberty and menopause, and well-woman care; (2) we need to increase the number of midwives so that all women can be served; and (3) we need systemic changes in the way health care is delivered in this country. Underlying all these is their understanding of the deep need for a change in how women and birth are viewed in this country. Jeannine Parvati Baker says that we need to remove the "mind swaddling" so that women can reconnect to their bodies and "re-member," as Candace Whitridge puts it, their ancient knowledge of how to birth. Midwifery can serve to reverse the progression of the technologization of birth in this country by striving to change what Penny Armstrong sees as more of a threat to birth than any laws: the dangerous "cultural imperative to separate us from the earth, from which

we get all our powers, and from our animal instincts." This ecofeminist theme of interconnection spirals from the individual act of a mother birthing her child to the community's responsibility in creating a sustainable future for the earth.

To build a sustainable future for midwifery I see the importance of building bridges between diverse groups who share a vision of the midwifery model of care. Connie Breece insists that midwives need time to organize and that they need to support each other in doing so. Potentially, midwives who have worked within different paradigms of midwifery are ideally situated to create a bridge between the "two different arms of midwifery" (as Fran Ventre put it) and work in partnership with women who want midwifery care accessible to them. Birthing women and midwifery activists need to be the driving force to keep the dialogue going between adversarial groups of midwives, keeping the aim on the common goals and good for midwifery and the women served by it. This philosophy of interconnection is articulated by midwife Caroline Flint:

> Midwives and women are intertwined; whatever affects women affects midwives and vice versa—we are interrelated and interwoven. When midwives are strong, women can labor safely and without interference. When midwives are weak, women's bodies are taken over and the birth process is interfered with, often to the detriment of women. (Flint 1987:4)

Keeping women central to the discussion and the political work needed to create a viable midwifery system of care in the United States is vital. Women and midwives working as partners have proven to be a powerful lobbying effort, as has been seen in New Zealand, Ontario, and England—all places in which independent midwifery has been integrated into the health care system.

A collaborative position paper from four of the major women's health care advocacy groups in the United States (Boston Women's Health Book Collective, National Black Women's Health Project, National Women's Health Network, and Women's Institute for Childbearing Policy) combines a philosophy of midwifery care designed to meet the needs of women and children with a public health perspective based on research and advocates the midwife as the person who most consistently can offer this comprehensive kind of care for women (Women's Institute for Childbearing Policy 1994). We can see the seeds of other cooperative efforts in the recent work of the Coalition for Improving Maternity Services (CIMS), which has documented

a vision and a plan calling for changes in maternal and child health care in the United States based on a midwifery model of care. A national consumer support organization, Citizens for Midwifery (CfM) has been born, and the boards of MANA and the ACNM, although still unable to work cooperatively, are at least in dialogue as they each strive to secure a future for the disparate visions of midwifery they hold.

Given the present rapid changes in the American health care system, it seems about as impossible to predict the future of midwifery as to successfully predict what a woman's labor will be like and how long it will last. I have always answered inquiries about labor predictions with, "It's not in my job description," claiming instead that a midwife's role is to encourage and be with a woman through the birth process in whatever way it unfolds for her. I can, however, share a personal vision of what I would *like* to see happen with midwifery, guided by the work done by many others. Just as visualization can help a woman imagine the process of giving birth and create positive pathways for a birth experience of her choice, creating a vision can help guide and mold the future of a profession. In retrospect we can see how *The Vision* (Association of Radical Midwives 1986), in Great Britain, demonstrates the influence of articulating a powerful vision. Ten years later that country is now engaged in radically revamping its maternal and child health care system.

Envisioning my own ideal practice of midwifery, I would like to be the community midwife, serving my immediate area (right now it covers an hour-drive radius). A local licensing board would recognize, regulate, discipline, and support me as an autonomous professional working in collaboration with physicians and health care providers of various health care modalities. Effective and respectful plans for transfer of care would be developed, with a mandatory provision of emergency and collaborative services to midwives and their clients. The regulating (licensing) boards would be public entities representing those who receive midwifery care, midwives, and other health care professionals.

I see a birth center central to that community, a place for women and families to gather for information, support, and health care. Those women who are at high risk and need medical care with an obstetrician could still maintain a link with the community birth center as a place of support. Breastfeeding support groups, parenting support groups, and other forms of related health care (herbal, nutrition, massage, etc.) are ongoing in the center. Women who choose homebirth also use the birth center as a place for community contact and support. As the community midwife I share a practice

with another midwife, and we attend to women in the place that they choose to birth. We have a small enough caseload to have a relationship with each of the birthing women and their families, time to do follow-up care in their homes. We refer the woman for special care when required, accessing extensive and diverse resources in the community. For example, I send a woman who is facing sexual abuse issues from her past to a counselor who helps her with those issues, and I refer her to a local support group. Simultaneously, I continue her care, helping her to integrate this new knowledge into her experience of pregnancy and birth. I refer a diabetic woman for more medical care and follow her progress, and still attend her birth in a hospital setting, in a collaborative management role. The birth center has massage therapists and other nonallopathic practitioners on hand, to give women the choice and chance to use different modalities of healing depending on their values and their unique needs. The birth center is multigenerational and provides a place for new and older mothers to share information and support.

I would include (as I do now) an apprentice in my practice who would gradually gain knowledge and increased responsibility as she witnesses and participates in the birth process. She would teach the childbirth classes and provide labor support, in turn learning from women the many ways that the birth process unfolds. Her educational process fits into a midwifery philosophy of holism, one that respects the connection between the caregiver, her apprentice, and the birthing mother. Learning, therefore, becomes integrated into the service of what is primary at birth—the experience of the mother and family. By learning from being at birth first, the natural authority and wisdom of birth is imparted before theoretical education dissects the process into parts. The apprentice supplements her experiential education with theoretical study available through a community-based program. When midwives are trained locally to serve the women in their communities, they are primarily accountable not to an institution but to the women and families in that community—as I am now. Other types of midwifery programs would be available as well, to serve the diversity of women who want to enter midwifery and work in the settings in which they feel most comfortable, adept, and supported.

This dream I know could be a reality—some of it is already true in my own practice and in some places in the world. For example, Holland incorporates several of these attributes in its system of midwifery care, and midwives in Ontario, Canada, working together with consumers, have designed such a system. As a result, today in Ontario there is a ratio of four women who have

to be turned away to every woman served, because there are not yet enough midwives to meet the demand for their services. This shows that limiting the government-approved ways in which midwives can be educated, as has been done in Ontario, seriously hinders their accessibility.

I have watched these other midwives organize and am compelled to spend more time midwifing the survival and growth of midwifery as a whole than midwifing individual women. At present I am putting my energy into creating diverse routes of entry to midwifery education on a national and local level so that midwives can stay and serve in their own communities. And I work to preserve our heritage of midwifery by collecting MANA's history in archival form for present and future historians, so that they will be able to retrace the renaissance of midwifery in North America. I want to continue to bring midwives' stories and visions to light, honoring and recognizing their work serving women in childbirth all over our country today. And I am trying to take the lessons I've learned in birth and use them in my organizational work in the world.

Most important, I want to be able to continue working with women in a way that allows me to have a relationship with them. For me this is the essence of midwifery, both in what I can give and what I receive. A relationship acknowledges that the effects are felt both ways. When a woman gives birth after a hard labor that challenges her to her core, the courage and grace she finds to help her are something I can share and be rewarded with if I am present and deeply connected. And because I personally know the mothers and families in my community, not only do they receive the satisfaction of personalized continuity of care, but I reap the rewards of seeing them grow through the birth process and watching their children grow and in turn having children. This is a reward that many midwives, especially those who work in hospitals, do not receive.

The sisterhood and support I find from birthing women and other midwives are also what sustains me in the wake of fear, grief, and uncertainty. Since I am not in jail, as some midwives are for their commitment and service, nor have I been burned at the stake for heresy or forced into silence and separation, I strive to make that true for all midwives who practice today.

The three strands of midwives come from different historical roots; they have often existed side-by-side or miles apart. As sisters in this journey we are now beginning to intertwine them to form a braid far stronger than each alone. The strength of this braid will come from the union of these different perspectives, each with its own integrity, wisdom, and unique history. The

strength of the grand midwife is her history and connection to the past, as she hands down women's wisdom and trust in the natural process in an unbroken chain. The nurse-midwife has increased the validity and power of midwifery within the current health care system and nurtured the links to medicine, essential to the provision of full-spectrum care. The independent midwife reminds us of our allegiance to women, to homebirth, and to midwifery as an autonomous profession that honors and respects the wisdom of women's bodies and sets its own standards for their care.

If we can reverse the direction of isolation and separation that has been the hallmark of the history of midwifery in the United States and move toward connection—connection between mind and body, mother and child, midwife and family, and family and community, as well as among the three strands of midwifery—midwifery will not only survive but will flourish. If I choose to look for and see unity in mind and body, in my many selves, and in my profession, I come to a place of peace. Just as diverse shapes and colors can create a pattern of harmony and beauty, so can midwives and women work together to weave a tapestry of effective and empowering care that will last for generations, preserving the joint legacies of today's midwives for the children of the future.

Appendix A

MANA Statement of Values and Ethics

We, as midwives, have a responsibility to educate ourselves and others regarding our values and ethics and reflect them in our practices. Our exploration of ethical midwifery is a critical reflection on moral issues as they pertain to maternal/child health on every level. This statement is intended to provide guidance for professional conduct in the practice of midwifery, as well as for MANA's policy making, thereby promoting quality care for childbearing families. MANA recognizes this document as an open, ongoing articulation of our evolution regarding values and ethics.

First, we recognize that values often go unstated, and yet our ethics (how we act) proceed directly from a foundation of values. Since what we hold precious, that is, what we value, infuses and informs our ethical decisions and actions, the Midwives' Alliance of North America wished explicitly to affirm our values as follows:[1]

I. *Woman as an Individual with Unique Value and Worth:*

A. We value women and their creative, life-affirming and life-giving powers which find expression in a diversity of ways.

B. We value a woman's right to make choices regarding all aspects of her life.

---

1. The membership largely agrees with the values that follow. However, some may word them differently or may leave out a few. This document is written to prompt personal reflection and clarification, not to represent absolute opinions.

Source: MANA, P.O. Box 175, Newton, KS 67114, (316) 283-4543. Reproduced by permission.

II. *Mother and Baby as Whole:*

A. We value the oneness of the pregnant mother and her unborn child—an inseparable and interdependent whole.

B. We value the birth experience as a rite of passage; the sentient and sensitive nature of the newborn; and the right of each baby to be born in a caring and loving manner, without separation from mother and family.

C. We value the integrity of a woman's body to be totally supported in her efforts to achieve a natural, spontaneous vaginal birth.

D. We value the breastfeeding relationship as the ideal way of nourishing and nurturing the newborn.

III. *The Nature of Birth:*

A. We value the essential mystery of birth.[2]

B. We value pregnancy and birth as natural processes that technology will never supplant.[3]

C. We value the integrity of life's experiences; the physical, emotional, mental, psychological and spiritual components of a process are inseparable.

D. We value pregnancy and birth as personal, intimate, internal,[4] sexual and social events to be shared in the environment and with the attendants a woman chooses.

E. We value the learning experiences of life and birth.

F. We value pregnancy and birth as processes which have lifelong impact on a woman's self-esteem, her health, her ability to nurture, and her personal growth.

IV. *The Art of Midwifery:*

A. We value our right to practice the art of midwifery. We value our work as an ancient vocation of women which has existed as long as humans have lived on earth.

B. We value expertise which incorporates academic knowledge, clinical skill, intuitive judgment and spiritual awareness.[5]

C. We value all forms of midwifery education and acknowledge the ongoing wisdom of apprenticeship as the original model for training midwives.

---

2. *Mystery* is defined as something that has not been or cannot be explained or understood; the quality or state of being incomprehensible or inexplicable; a tenet which cannot be understood in terms of human reason.

3. *Supplant* means to supersede by force or cunning; to take the place of.

4. In this context *internal* refers to the fact that birth happens within the body and psyche of the woman. Ultimately she and only she can give birth.

5. An expert is one whose knowledge and skill is specialized and profound, especially as the result of practical experience.

D. We value the art of nurturing the intrinsic normalcy of birth and recognize that each woman and baby has parameters of well-being unique unto themselves.

E. We value the empowerment of women in all aspects of life and particularly as that strength is realized during pregnancy, birth and thereafter. We value the art of encouraging the open expression of that strength so women can birth unhindered and confident in their abilities and in our support.

F. We value skills which support a complicated pregnancy or birth to move toward a state of greater well-being or to be brought to the most healing conclusion possible. We value the art of letting go.[6]

G. We value the acceptance of death as a possible outcome of birth. We value our focus as supporting life rather than avoiding death.[7]

H. We value standing for what we believe in the face of social and political oppression.

V. *Woman as Mother:*

A. We value a mother's intuitive knowledge of herself and her baby before, during and after birth.[8]

B. We value a woman's innate ability to nurture her pregnancy and birth her baby; the power and beauty of her body as it grows and the awesome strength summoned in labor.

C. We value the mother as the only direct care provider for her unborn child.[9]

D. We value supporting women in a nonjudgmental way, whatever their state of physical, emotional, social or spiritual health. We value the broadening of available resources whenever possible so that the desired

---

6. This addresses our desire for an uncomplicated birth whenever possible and recognizes that there are times when it is not possible. For example, due to problems with the birth, a woman may be least traumatized to have a surgical delivery. If a spontaneous vaginal birth is not possible, then we let go of that goal in order to achieve the possibility of a healthy mother and baby. Likewise, the situation where parents choose to allow a very ill, premature or deformed infant to die in their arms rather than being subjected to multiple surgeries, separations and ICU stays. This too, is a letting go of the normal for the most healing choice possible within the framework of the parents' ethics given the circumstances. What is most healing will, of course, vary from individual to individual.

7. We place the emphasis of our care on supporting life (preventive measures, good nutrition, emotional health, etc.) and not pathology, diagnosis, treatment of problems, and heroic solutions in an attempt to preserve life at any cost of quality.

8. This addresses the medical model's tendency to ignore a woman's sense of well-being or danger in many aspects of health care, but particularly in regard to her pregnancy.

9. This acknowledges that the thrust of our care centers on the mother, her health, her well-being, her nutrition, her habits, her emotional balance, and, in turn, the baby benefits. This view is diametrically opposed to the medical model, which often attempts to care for the fetus/baby while dismissing or even excluding the mother.

goals of health, happiness and personal growth are realized according to their needs and perceptions.

E. We value the right of each woman to choose a caregiver appropriate to her needs and compatible with her belief systems.

F. We value pregnancy and birth as rites of passage integral to a woman's evolution into mothering.

G. We value the potential of partners, family and community to support women in all aspects of birth and mothering.[10]

VI. *The Nature of Relationship:*

A. We value relationship. The quality, integrity, equality and uniqueness of our interactions inform and critique our choices and decisions.

B. We value honesty in relationship.

C. We value caring for women to the best of our ability without prejudice against their age, race, religion, culture, sexual orientation, physical abilities, or socioeconomic background.

D. We value the concept of personal responsibility and the right of individuals to make choices regarding what they deem best for themselves. We value the right to true informed choice, not merely informed consent to what we think is best.

E. We value our relationship to a process larger than ourselves, recognizing that birth is something we can seek to learn from and know, but never control.

F. We value humility in our work.

G. We value the recognition of our own limits and limitations.

H. We value direct access to information readily understood by all.

I. We value sharing information and our understanding about birth experiences, skills, and knowledge.

J. We value the midwifery community as a support system and an essential place of learning and sisterhood.

K. We value diversity among midwives; recognizing that it broadens our collective resources and challenges us to work for greater understanding of birth and each other.

L. We value mutual trust and respect, which grows from a realization of all of the above.

Making Decisions and Acting Ethically

These values reflect our feelings regarding how we frame midwifery in our hearts and minds. However, due to the broad range of geographic, religious, cultural, political, educational, and personal backgrounds among our membership, how

---

10. While partners, other family members, and a woman's larger community can and often do provide her with vital support, in using the word *potential* we wish to acknowledge that many women find themselves pregnant and mothering in abusive or otherwise unsafe environments.

we act based on these values will be very individual. Acting ethically is a complex merging of our values and these background influences combined with the relationship we have to others who may be involved in the process taking place. We call upon all these resources when deciding how to respond in the moment to each situation.

We acknowledge the limitations of ethical codes which present a list of rules which must be followed, recognizing that such a code may interfere with, rather than enhance, our ability to make choices. To apply such rules we must have moral integrity, an ability to make judgments, and we must have adequate information; with all of these an appeal to a code becomes superfluous. Furthermore, when we set up rigid ethical codes we may begin to cease considering the transformations we go through as a result of our choices as well as negate our wish to foster truly diversified practice. Rules are not something we can appeal to when all else fails. However, this is the illusion fostered by traditional codes of ethics.[11] MANA's support of the individual's moral integrity grows out of an understanding that there cannot possibly be one right answer for all situations.

We acknowledge the following basic concepts and believe that ethical judgments can be made with these thoughts in mind:

- Moral agency and integrity are born within the heart of each individual.
- Judgments are fundamentally based on awareness and understanding of ourselves and others and are primarily derived from one's own sense of moral integrity with reference to clearly articulated values. Becoming aware and increasing our understanding are ongoing processes facilitated by our efforts at personal growth on every level. The wisdom gained by this process cannot be taught or dictated, but one can learn to realize, experience and evaluate it.
- The choices one can or will actually make may be limited by the oppressive nature of the medical, legal or cultural framework in which we live. The more our values conflict with those of the dominant culture, the more risky it becomes to act truly in accord with our values.
- The pregnant woman and midwife are both individual moral agents unique unto themselves, having independent value and worth.

We support both midwives and the women and families we serve to follow and make known the dictates of our own conscience as our relationship begins, evolves and especially when decisions must be made which impact us or the care being provided. It is up to us to work out a mutually satisfactory relationship when and if that is possible.

It is useful to understand the two basic theories upon which moral judgments and decision-making processes are based. These processes become particularly important when one considers that in our profession, a given woman's rights may

---

11. Hoagland, Sarah, paraphrased from her book *Lesbian Ethics*.

not be absolute in all cases, or that in certain situations the woman may not be considered autonomous or competent to make her own decision.

One of the main theories of ethics states that one should look to the consequences of the act (*i.e.,* the outcome) and not the act itself to determine if it is appropriate care. This point of view looks for the greatest good for the greatest number. The other primary ethical theory states that one should look to the act itself (*i.e.,* type of care provided) and if it is right, then this could override the net outcome. This is a more process-oriented, feminist perspective. Midwives weave these two perspectives in the process of making decisions in their practice. Since the outcome of pregnancy is ultimately an unknown and is always unknowable, it is inevitable that in certain circumstances our best decisions in the moment will lead to consequences we could not foresee.

In summary, acting ethically is facilitated by:

- Carefully defining our values.
- Weighing the values in consideration with those of the community of midwives, families, and culture in which we find ourselves.
- Acting in accord with our values to the best or our ability as the situation demands.
- Engaging in ongoing self-examination and evaluation.

There are both individual and social implications to any decision-making process. The actual roles and oppressive aspects of a society are never exact, and therefore conflicts may arise, and we must weigh which choices or obligations take precedence over others. There are inevitably times when resolution does not occur and we cannot make peace with any course of action or may feel conflicted about a choice already made. The community of women, both midwives and those we serve, will provide a fruitful resource for continued moral support and guidance.

Bibliography: Cross, Star, MANA Ethics Chair, 1989, unpublished draft of ethics code. Daly, Mary, *Gynecology: The Metaethics of Radical Feminism,* Beacon Press, Boston, MA, 1978. Hoagland, Sarah Lucia, *Lesbian Ethics: Toward New Value,* Institute of Lesbian Studies, Palo Alto, CA, 1988. Johnson, Sonia, *Going Out of Our Minds: The Metaphysics of Liberation,* Crossing Press, Freedom, CA, 1987.

Appendix B

CIMS Document: The Mother-Friendly Childbirth Initiative

Mission

The Coalition for Improving Maternity Services (CIMS) is a coalition of individuals and national organizations with concern for the care and well-being of mothers, babies, and families. Our mission is to promote a wellness model of maternity care that will improve birth outcomes and substantially reduce costs. This evidence-based mother-, baby- and family-friendly model focuses on prevention and wellness as the alternatives to high-cost screening, diagnosis, and treatment programs.

Preamble

Whereas:

- In spite of spending far more money per capita on maternity and newborn care than any other country, the United States falls behind most industrialized countries in perinatal morbidity and mortality, and maternal mortality is four times greater for African-American women than for Euro-American women;
- Midwives attend the vast majority of births in those industrialized countries with the best perinatal outcomes, yet in the United States, midwives are the principal attendants at only a small percentage of births;

Source: The First Consensus Initiative of the Coalition for Improving Maternity Services (CIMS). Copyright 1996 by the Coalition for Improving Maternity Services (CIMS), POB 382724, Cambridge, MA 02238. Permission granted to freely reproduce in whole or in part with complete attribution.

- Current maternity and newborn practices that contribute to high costs and inferior outcomes include the inappropriate application of technology and routine procedures that are not based on scientific evidence;
- Increased dependence on technology has diminished confidence in women's innate ability to give birth without intervention;
- The integrity of the mother-child relationship, which begins in pregnancy, is compromised by the obstetrical treatment of mother and baby as if they were separate units with conflicting needs;
- Although breastfeeding has been scientifically shown to provide optimum health, nutritional, and developmental benefits to newborns and their mothers, only a fraction of U.S. mothers are fully breastfeeding their babies by the age of six weeks;
- The current maternity care system in the United States does not provide equal access to health care resources for women from disadvantaged population groups, women without insurance, and women whose insurance dictates caregivers or place of birth;

Therefore:

We, the undersigned members of CIMS, hereby resolve to define and promote mother-friendly maternity services in accordance with the following principles:

Principles

We believe the philosophical cornerstones of mother-friendly care to be as follows:

Normalcy of the Birthing Process

- Birth is a normal, natural, and healthy process.
- Women and babies have the inherent wisdom necessary for birth.
- Babies are aware, sensitive human beings at the time of birth and should be acknowledged and treated as such.
- Breastfeeding provides the optimum nourishment for newborns and infants.
- Birth can safely take place in hospitals, birth centers, and homes.
- The midwifery model of care, which supports and protects the normal birth process, is the most appropriate for the majority of women during pregnancy and birth.

Empowerment

- A woman's confidence and ability to give birth and to care for her baby are enhanced or diminished by every person who gives her care, and by the environment in which she gives birth.
- A mother and baby are distinct yet interdependent during pregnancy, birth, and infancy. Their interconnectedness is vital and must be respected.

- Pregnancy, birth, and the postpartum period are milestone events in the continuum of life. These experiences profoundly affect women, babies, fathers, and families, and have important and long-lasting effects on society.

Autonomy

Every woman should have the opportunity to:
- Have a healthy and joyous birth experience for herself and her family, regardless of her age or circumstances;
- Give birth as she wishes in an environment in which she feels nurtured and secure, and her emotional well-being, privacy, and personal preferences are respected;
- Have access to the full range of options for pregnancy, birth, and nurturing her baby, and to accurate information on all available birthing sites, caregivers, and practices;
- Receive accurate and up-to-date information about the benefits and risks of all procedures, drugs, and tests suggested for use during pregnancy, birth, and the postpartum period, with the rights to informed consent and informed refusal;
- Receive support for making informed choices about what is best for her and her baby based on her individual values and beliefs.

Do No Harm

- Interventions should not be applied routinely during pregnancy, birth, or the postpartum period. Many standard medical tests, procedures, technologies, and drugs carry risks to both mother and baby and should be avoided in the absence of specific scientific indications for their use.
- If complications arise during pregnancy, birth, or the postpartum period, medical treatments should be evidence-based.

Responsibility

- Each caregiver is responsible for the quality of care she or he provides.
- Maternity care practice should be based not on the needs of the caregiver or provider, but solely on the needs of the mother and child.
- Each hospital and birth center is responsible for the periodic review and evaluation, according to current scientific evidence, of the effectiveness, risks, and rates of use of its medical procedures for mothers and babies.
- Society, through both its government and the public health establishment, is responsible for ensuring access to maternity services for all women and for monitoring the quality of those services.
- Individuals are ultimately responsible for making informed choices about the health care they and their babies receive.

These principles give rise to the following steps which support, protect, and promote mother-friendly maternity services:

Ten Steps of the Mother-Friendly Childbirth Initiative for Mother-Friendly Hospitals, Birth Centers, and Home Birth Services

To receive CIMS designation as "mother-friendly," a hospital, birth center, or home birth service must carry out the above philosophical principles by fulfilling the Ten Steps of Mother-Friendly Care:

A Mother-Friendly hospital, birth center, or home birth service:

1. Offers all birthing mothers:
   - Unrestricted access to the birth companions of her choice, including fathers, partners, children, family members, and friends;
   - Unrestricted access to continuous emotional and physical support from a skilled woman—for example, a doula [labor-support professional];
   - Access to professional midwifery care.
2. Provides accurate descriptive and statistical information to the public about its practices and procedures for birth care, including measures of interventions and outcomes.
3. Provides culturally competent care—that is, care that is sensitive and responsive to the specific beliefs, values, and customs of the mother's ethnicity and religion.
4. Provides the birthing woman with the freedom to walk, move about, and assume the positions of her choice during labor and birth (unless restriction is specifically required to correct a complication) and discourages the use of the lithotomy (flat on back with legs elevated) position.
5. Has clearly defined policies and procedures for:
   - Collaborating and consulting throughout the perinatal period with other maternity services, including communicating with the original caregiver when transfer from one birth site to another is necessary;
   - Linking the mother and baby to appropriate community resources, including prenatal and postdischarge follow-up and breastfeeding support.
6. Does not routinely employ practices and procedures that are unsupported by scientific evidence, including but not limited to the following:
   - shaving;
   - enemas;
   - IVs (intravenous drip);
   - withholding nourishment;
   - early rupture of membranes;
   - electronic fetal monitoring.

Other interventions are limited as follows:
- Has an oxytocin use rate of 10% or less for induction and augmentation;
- Has an episiotomy rate of 20% or less, with a goal of 5% or less;
- Has a total cesarean rate of 10% or less in community hospitals, and 15% or less in tertiary-care (high-risk) hospitals;
- Has a VBAC (vaginal birth after cesarean) rate of 60% or more with a goal of 75% or more.

7. Educates staff in non-drug methods of pain relief and does not promote the use of analgesic or anesthetic drugs not specifically required to correct a complication.
8. Encourages all mothers and families, including those with sick or premature newborns or infants with congenital problems, to touch, hold, breastfeed, and care for their babies to the extent compatible with their conditions.
9. Discourages non-religious circumcision of the newborn.
10. Strives to achieve the WHO-UNICEF "Ten Steps of the Baby-Friendly Hospital Initiative" to promote successful breastfeeding:
    1. Have a written breastfeeding policy communicated to all health care staff;
    2. Train all health care staff in skills necessary to implement this policy;
    3. Inform all pregnant women about the benefits and management of breastfeeding;
    4. Help mothers initiate breastfeeding within a half-hour of birth;
    5. Show mothers how to breastfeed and how to maintain lactation even if they should be separated from their infants;
    6. Give newborn infants no food or drink other than breast milk unless medically indicated;
    7. Practice rooming in: allow mothers and infants to remain together 24 hours a day;
    8. Encourage breastfeeding on demand;
    9. Give no artificial teat or pacifiers (also called dummies or soothers) to breastfeeding infants;
    10. Foster the establishment of breastfeeding support groups and refer mothers to them on discharge from hospitals or clinics.

Bibliography

"ACOG Official: Home Delivery Maternal Trauma, Child Abuse." *Obstetrics and Gynecology News* (October 1, 1977): 1.

American College of Nurse-Midwives (ACNM) Board of Directors. "The ACNM Position Statement on Midwifery Education." *Journal of Nurse-Midwifery* 41,5 (September/October 1996): 354.

Anderson, Rondi E., and Patricia Aikins Murphy. "Outcomes of 11,788 Planned Home Births Attended by Certified Nurse-Midwives: A Retrospective Descriptive Study." *Journal of Nurse-Midwifery* 40,6 (November/December 1995): 483–492.

Arms, Suzanne. *Immaculate Deception*. New York: Bantam Books, 1975.

———. *Creating a Sustainable Future in Midwifery*. Audiotape from the MANA conference, Phoenix, Ariz., 1995.

Armstrong, Penny, and Sheryl Feldman. *A Midwife's Story*. New York: Arbor House, 1986.

———. *A Wise Birth*. New York: Morrow, 1990.

Arney, William R. *Power and the Profession of Obstetrics*. Chicago: University of Chicago Press, 1982.

Association of Radical Midwives (ARM). *The Vision: Proposals for the Future of the Maternity Services*. ARM, 62 Greetby Hill, Ormskirk, Lancashire, United Kingdom L39 2DT, 1986.

Belenky, Mary, Blythe Clinchy, Nancy Goldberger, and Jill Tarule. *Women's Ways of Knowing: The Development of Self, Voice, and Mind*. New York: Basic Books, 1986.

Bennett, Ruth. "Midwifery Careers and Continuing Education." In *Proceedings of*

the International Confederation of Midwives Twenty-third International Congress 1 (1993): 177.

Bergum, Vangie. *Woman to Mother: A Transformation.* South Hadley, Mass.: Bergin and Garvey, 1989.

Bortin, Sylvia, Marina Alzugaray, Judy Dowd, and Janice Kalman. "A Feminist Perspective on the Study of Home Birth: Application of a Midwifery Care Framework." *Journal of Nurse-Midwifery* 39,3 (1994): 142–149.

Boston Women's Health Book Collective. *Our Bodies, Ourselves: A Book by and for Women,* 2d ed. New York: Simon and Schuster, 1979.

Bovard, Wendy, and Gladys Milton. *Why Not Me Lord? The Story of Gladys Milton, Midwife.* Summertown, Tenn.: Book Publishing Co., 1993.

Bowland, Kate, Peggy Spindel, and Fran Ventre. "The Transition from Lay Midwife to Certified Nurse-Midwife in the United States." *Journal of Nurse-Midwifery* 40,5 (1995): 428–437.

Boyer, Ernest. "Midwifery in America: A Profession Reaffirmed." *Journal of Nurse-Midwifery* 35,4 (1990): 214–219.

Breckinridge, Mary. *Wide Neighborhoods: A Story of the Frontier Nursing Service.* Lexington: University Press of Kentucky, 1981.

Burnett, C., J. Jones, J. Rooks, C. Tyler, and A. Miller. "Home Delivery and Neonatal Mortality in North Carolina." *Journal of the American Medical Association* 244,24 (1980): 2741–2745.

Burst, Helen Varney. "'Real' Midwifery." *Journal of Nurse-Midwifery* 35,4 (November/December 1990): 189.

———. "An Update on the Credentialing of Midwives by the ACNM." *Journal of Nurse-Midwifery* 40,3 (1995): 290.

Burst, Helen Varney, and Anne T. Vosler. "Nurse-Midwifery as It Reinforces and Transforms the American Ideology of Gender Roles." *Journal of Nurse-Midwifery* 38,5 (September/October 1993): 293.

Buss, Fran Leeper. *La Partera: Story of a Midwife.* Ann Arbor: University of Michigan Press, 1980.

Campbell, Marie. *Folks Do Get Born.* New York: Rinehart, 1946.

Coalition for Improving Maternity Services (CIMS). "The Mother-Friendly Initiative." CIMS, P.O. Box 382724, Cambridge, Mass. 02238, 1996.

Coalition of Ontario Midwifery and Birth Schools (COMBS). *Newsletter* (Summer 1992): 11–19. COMBS, Box 3924, Station C, Ottawa, Ontario K1Y 4M5, Canada.

Cohen, Nancy Wainer. *Open Season: Survival Guide for Natural Childbirth and VBAC in the '90s.* New York: Bergin and Garvey, 1991.

Cohen, Nancy Wainer, and Lois Estner. *Silent Knife: Cesarean Prevention and Vaginal Birth after Cesarean.* South Hadley, Mass.: Bergin and Garvey, 1983.

Davis, Elizabeth. *Heart and Hands: A Midwife's Guide to Pregnancy and Birth.* Berkeley, Calif.: Celestial Arts, 1987.

————. "Women's Ways of Knowing." Lecture presented at MANA conference, New York, 1992.

Davis, Elizabeth, and Robbie Davis-Floyd. "Intuition as Authoritative Knowledge in Midwifery and Homebirth." In "The Social Production of Authoritative Knowledge in Childbirth," a special issue of the *Medical Anthropology Quarterly,* new series 10,2 (1996): 237–269, Robbie Davis-Floyd and Carolyn Sargent, guest editors.

Davis-Floyd, Robbie. *Birth as an American Rite of Passage.* Berkeley: University of California Press, 1992.

————. "The Technocratic Body: American Childbirth as Cultural Expression." *Social Science Medicine* 38,8 (1994): 1125–1140.

Davis-Putt, Betty Anne, et al. "Submission to CDC Calling for Community-based Midwifery through Regional Schools." *COMBS* (Coalition of Ontario Midwifery and Birth Schools) *Newsletter* 1,1 (1992): 11–18.

Decker, Barbara. "Implementation of the Mastery Learning/Modular Curriculum in Nurse Midwifery Education." *Journal of Nurse-Midwifery* 35,1 (January/February 1990): 3–9.

DeClercq, Eugene. "Politics, Midwifery, and the Law: A Cross-National Perspective." In *Proceedings of the International Confederation of Midwives Twenty-third International Congress* 1 (1993): 529–540.

DeLee, Joseph B. "The Prophylactic Forceps Operation." *American Journal of Obstetrics and Gynecology* 1 (1920): 34–44.

Devitt, Neal. "The Transition from Home to Hospital Birth in the U.S." *Birth and the Family Journal* 4,1 (1977): 47–58.

DeVries, Raymond. *Regulating Birth: Midwives, Medicine, and the Law.* Philadelphia: Temple University Press, 1985.

————. "Barriers to Midwifery: An International Perspective." *Journal of Perinatal Education* 1. Washington, D.C.: American Society for Psychoprophylaxis in Obstetrics, 1992.

Dick-Read, Grantly. *Childbirth without Fear.* New York: Harper and Row, 1959.

Duden, Barbara. *Disembodying Women: Perspectives on Pregnancy and the Unborn.* Cambridge, Mass.: Harvard University Press, 1993.

Durand, A. Mark. "The Safety of Home Birth: The Farm Study." *American Journal of Public Health* 82,3 (1992): 450–453.

Eakins, Pamela, ed. *The American Way of Birth.* Philadelphia: Temple University Press, 1986.

Edwards, Margot, and Mary Waldorf. *Reclaiming Birth: History and Heroines of Childbirth Reform.* New York: Crossing Press, 1984.

Ehrenreich, Barbara, and Deirdre English. *Witches, Midwives, and Nurses: A History of Women Healers.* New York: Feminist Press, 1973.

Engleman, George. *Labor among Primitive Peoples.* New York: AMS Press, 1977.

Expert Maternity Group. *Changing Childbirth.* London: HMSO, 1995.

Flint, Caroline. *Sensitive Midwifery.* London: Heinemann, 1987.

Gaskin, Ina May. *Spiritual Midwifery,* rev. ed. Summertown, Tenn.: Book Publishing Co., 1978.

———. "Intuition and the Emergence of Authoritative Knowledge." *Medical Anthropology Quarterly* 10,2 (June 1996): 295–298.

Goer, Henci. *Obstetric Myths vs. Research Realities: A Guide to the Medical Literature.* Westport, Conn.: Bergin and Garvey, 1995.

Guilliland, Karen. "Professionalism vs. Partnership: Midwives and Women Hear the Heartbeat of the Future." In *Proceedings of the International Confederation of Midwives Twenty-third International Congress* 2 (1993): 784–789.

Hartley, Carla. *Helping Hands: The Apprentice Workbook.* Conroe, Tex.: Apprentice Academics, 1988.

Hinds, M., G. Bergeisen, and D. Allen. "Neonatal Outcome of Planned vs. Unplanned Out-of-Hospital Births in Kentucky." *Journal of the American Medical Association* 235,11 (1985): 1568–1582.

Hoff, G., and L. Schneiderman. "Having Babies at Home: Is It Safe? Is It Ethical?" *Hastings Center Report, Institute of Society, Ethics, and Life Science* (December 1985): 19–27.

Holmes, Linda Janet. "Thank You Jesus to Myself: The Life of a Traditional Black Midwife." In *The Black Women's Health Book: Speaking for Ourselves,* edited by Evelyn White. Seattle, Wash.: Seal Press, 1990.

Hubbard, Ruth. *The Politics of Women's Biology.* New Brunswick, N.J.: Rutgers University Press, 1992.

Jordan, Brigitte. *Birth in Four Cultures: A Cross-Cultural Investigation of Childbirth in Yucatan, Holland, Sweden, and the United States,* 4th ed. Prospect Heights, Ill.: Waveland Press, 1993.

Kahn, Robbie Pfeufer. *Bearing Meaning: The Language of Birth.* Chicago: University of Illinois Press, 1995.

Kirkham, Mavis. "Professionalism Past and Present: With Women or with the Powers That Be?" In *Midwifery Care for the Future,* edited by Debra Kroll. London: Balliere Tindall, 1996.

Kitzinger, Sheila. "Why Women Need Midwives." In *The Midwife Challenge,* edited by Sheila Kitzinger. London: Pandora Press, 1988.

Klaus, Marshall H., John Kennell, Gayle Berkowitz, and Phyllis Klaus. "Maternal Assistance and Support in Labor: Father, Nurse, Midwife, or Doula? *Clinical Consultations in Obstetrics and Gynecology* 4,4 (1992).

Leavitt, Judith. *Brought to Bed: Childbearing in America, 1750–1950.* New York: Oxford University Press, 1986.

Lichtman, Ronnie. "Medical Models and Midwifery: The Cultural Experience of Birth." In *Childbirth in America: Anthropological Perspectives,* edited by Karen Michaelson. South Hadley, Mass.: Bergin and Garvey, 1988.

———. "Entry-Level Degrees for Midwifery Practice." *Journal of Nurse-Midwifery* 41,1 (January/February 1996): 47–49.

Littoff, Judy, ed. *The American Midwife Debate: Sourcebook on Its Modern Origins.* Westport, Conn.: Greenwood Press, 1978.

Logan, Onnie Lee, as told to Katherine Clark. *Motherwit: An Alabama Midwife's Story*. New York: Dutton, 1989.

McKay, Susan. "Shared Power: The Essence of Humanized Childbirth." *Pre- and Peri-Natal Psychology Journal* 5,4 (1991): 283–296.

Martin, Emily. *The Woman in the Body: A Cultural Analysis of Reproduction*. Boston: Beacon Press, 1987.

Meadows, Jacqueline. Letter to the Editor. *Journal of Nurse-Midwifery* 32,4 (1987).

Mehl, Lewis, and Morgaine Mehl Madronna. "Future of Midwifery." *NAPSAC News* (Fall/Winter 1993/1994).

Mehl, Lewis, Gail Peterson, and M. Whitt. "Outcomes of Elective Home Births: A Series of 1146 Cases." *Journal of Reproductive Medicine* 19 (1977): 281–290.

Midwives' Alliance of North America (MANA). "Statement of Values and Ethics." *MANA News* 1992.

———. "Core Competencies." *MANA News* 1994.

Moran, Marilyn. *Birth and the Dialogue of Love*. Leawood, Kans.: New Nativity Press, 1981.

Morris, Donna L., et al. "How Much Intervention Is Enough? A Study of Low-Risk Certified Nurse-Midwife Managed Labor and Delivery Outcomes." In *Proceedings of the International Confederation of Midwives Twenty-third International Congress* 3 (1993): 1332–1339.

Murphy, Patricia. Editorial: "What Is a Nurse-Midwife?" *Journal of Nurse-Midwifery* 32,3 (1987): 121.

North American Registry of Midwives (NARM). Information packet, 1996.

Oakley, Ann. *Becoming a Mother*. New York: Schocken Books, 1980.

Page, Lesley. "Education for Practice." *MIDRS Midwifery Digest* 3,3 (1993): 253–256.

Rabuzzi, Kathryn Allen. *Mother with Child: Transformations through Childbirth*. Indianapolis: Indiana University Press, 1994.

Razak, Arizika. "Towards a Womanist Analysis of Birth." In *Reweaving the World: The Emergence of Ecofeminism*, edited by Irene Diamond and Gloria Feman Orenstein. San Francisco: Sierra Club Books, 1990.

Reichman, Sylvia. *Transitions*. Marble Hill, Mo.: National Association of Parents and Professionals for Safe Alternatives in Childbirth (NAPSAC) Reproductions, 1988.

Reid, Margaret. "Sisterhood and Professionalization: A Case Study of the American Lay Midwife." In *Women as Healers: Cross-Cultural Perspectives*, edited by Carol McClain. New Brunswick, N.J.: Rutgers University Press, 1989.

Rich, Adrienne. *Of Woman Born: Motherhood as Experience and Institution*. New York: Norton, 1976.

Roberts, Joyce. Editorial: "Professionalism and Nurse-Midwifery." *Journal of Nurse-Midwifery* 38,6 (1993): 321.

Rooks, Judith. *Childbearing in America: The Past, Present, and Potential Role of Midwives*. Philadelphia: Temple University Press, 1997.

Rooks, Judith P., and Katherine Camacho Carr. "Criteria for Accreditation of Direct-Entry Midwifery Education." *Journal of Nurse-Midwifery* 40,3 (1995): 297.

Rooks, Judith P., Norman L. Weatherby, Eunice Ernst, Susan Stapleton, David Rosen, and Allan Rosenfield. "Outcomes of Care in Birth Centers: The National Birth Center Study." *New England Journal of Medicine* 321 (1989): 1804–1811.

Rossiter, Amy. *From Private to Public: A Feminist Exploration of Early Mothering.* Toronto: Women's Press, 1988.

Rothman, Barbara Katz. *In Labor: Women and Power in the Birthplace.* New York: Norton, 1982.

———. *Re-creating Motherhood: Ideology and Technology in a Patriarchal Society.* New York: Norton, 1989.

———. *Midwifery: Who's Talking, Who's Listening?* Audiotape from the Massachusetts Friends of Midwives Conference, Boston, 1993.

Sakala, Carol. "Content of Care by Independent Midwives: Assistance with Pain in Labor and Birth." *Social Science and Medicine* 26,11 (1988): 1141–1158.

———. "Midwifery Care and Out-of-Hospital Birth Settings: How Do They Reduce Unnecessary Cesarean Births?" *Social Science Medicine* 37,10 (1993): 1233–1250.

Schlinger, Hilary. *Circle of Midwives.* New York: Schlinger, 1992.

Scoggin, Janet. "How Nurse-Midwives Define Themselves in Relation to Nursing, Medicine, and Midwifery." *Journal of Nurse-Midwifery* 41,1 (January/February 1996): 36–42.

Shanley, Laura Kaplan. *Unassisted Childbirth.* Westport, Conn.: Bergin and Garvey, 1994.

Silverton, Louise. "Educating for the Future." In *Midwifery Care for the Future: Meeting the Challenge.* London: Bailliere Tindall, 1996.

Smith, Margaret Charles, and Linda Janet Holmes. *Listen to Me Good: The Life Story of an Alabama Midwife.* Columbus: Ohio State University Press, 1996.

Starr, Paul. *The Social Transformation of Medicine.* New York: Basic Books, 1982.

Suarez, Suzanne. "Midwifery Is Not the Practice of Medicine." *Yale Journal of Law and Feminism* 5,2 (1993): 316–369.

Sullivan, Deborah, and Ruth Beeman. "Four Years' Experience with Home Birth by Licensed Midwives in Arizona." *Journal of the American Public Health Association* 73,6 (1983): 641–645.

Sullivan, Deborah, and Rose Weitz. *Labor Pains: Modern Midwives and Home Birth.* New Haven, Conn.: Yale University Press, 1988.

Susie, Debra Anne. *In the Way of Our Grandmothers: A Cultural View of Twentieth-Century Midwifery in Florida.* Athens: University of Georgia Press, 1988.

Tew, Marjorie. *Safer Childbirth?: A Critical History of Maternity Care.* New York: Routledge, Chapman, and Hall, 1990.

Ulrich, Laurel. *Good Wives.* New York: Oxford University Press, 1982.

————. *A Midwife's Tale: The Life of Martha Ballard, Based on Her Diary, 1785–1812.* New York: Vintage Books, 1991.

United Kingdom. House of Commons. *Health Care Committee Report on Maternity Services.* London: HMSO, 1992.

Varney, Helen. *Nurse-Midwifery,* 2d ed. Boston: Blackwell Scientific, 1987.

Walsh, Linda. "Profession, Home-based Craft, or Spiritual Calling? Urban American Midwifery in the Early Twentieth Century." In *Proceedings of the International Confederation of Midwives Twenty-third Congress* 4 (1993): 1999–2010.

Walsh, Linda, and Ann Lyn Jaspan. "Lay Midwife to Nurse-Midwife: Perceived Learning Needs and Attitudes toward the Learning Experience." *Journal of Nurse-Midwifery* 35,4 (1990): 204–213.

Wellish, Pam, and Susan Root. *Hearts Open Wide: Midwives and Births.* Berkeley, Calif.: Wingbow Press, 1987.

Wertz, Richard, and Dorothy Wertz. *Lying-In: A History of Childbirth in America.* New Haven, Conn.: Yale University Press, 1989.

World Health Organization. "Appropriate Technology for Birth." *Lancet* (August 24, 1985): 436–437.

Women's Institute for Childbearing Policy. *Childbearing Policy within a National Health Program: An Evolving Consensus for New Directions.* Boston: Women's Institute for Childbearing Policy, 1994.

Index

(Page numbers in italics refer to photographs.)

About the Authors

Penfield Chester is a midwife with a rural homebirth practice in western Massachusetts. She has been attending births since 1980 and got involved in local and national midwifery organizational politics after her son was born in 1984. She is presently the New England regional representative and education committee chair of the Midwives' Alliance of North America. She has taught a course entitled "Current Politics of Birth and Midwifery" in local colleges and speaks on midwifery education. For two years she coordinated a midwifery program for aspiring midwives in New England. Her training as a massage therapist and hospice volunteer have expanded her approach to midwifery. She received her M.A. in women's studies with a focus in midwifery from the graduate program of Vermont College in 1995, and became a Certified Professional Midwife (CPM) in 1996.

Sarah Chester McKusick is the mother of three daughters, all of whose births were assisted by her sister Penfield Chester. Over the past twenty years she has traveled and photographed extensively in the United States, Asia, Europe, and Central America, being drawn to portraiture and documenting social landscapes. She and her daughters and husband live on an old New England farm in western Massachusetts.

78
5-98

161 TOL
FB
E-70

L339
8339
CLE

NORTHWESTERN
CONSERVATION, INC.

D0073439